be a
beautiful
bride

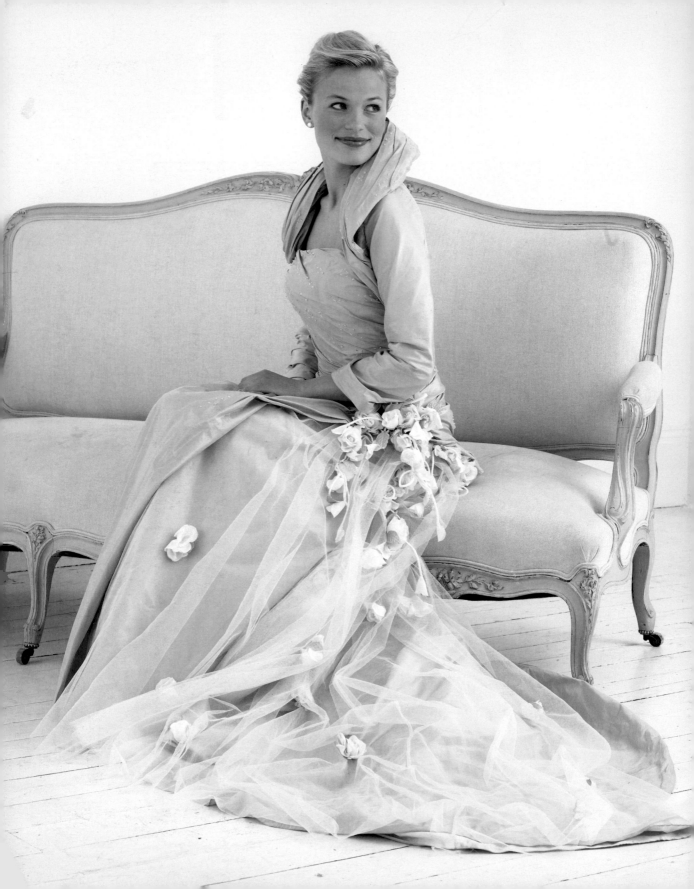

hamlyn

be a beautiful bride

Veronique Henderson
Pat Henshaw

with colour**me**beautiful

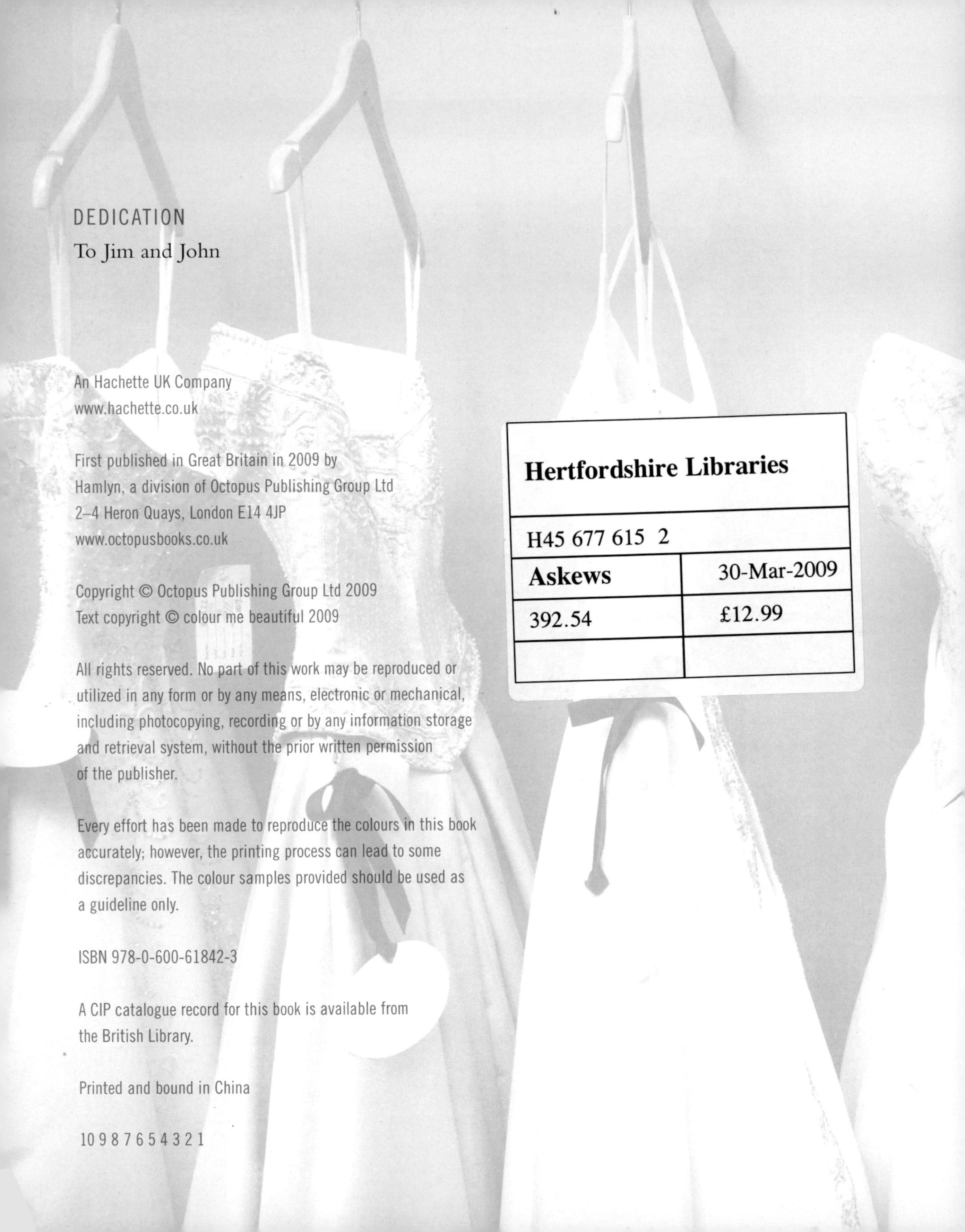

DEDICATION

To Jim and John

An Hachette UK Company
www.hachette.co.uk

First published in Great Britain in 2009 by
Hamlyn, a division of Octopus Publishing Group Ltd
2–4 Heron Quays, London E14 4JP
www.octopusbooks.co.uk

Every effort has been made to reproduce the colours in this book
accurately; however, the printing process can lead to some
discrepancies. The colour samples provided should be used as
a guideline only.

ISBN 978-0-600-61842-3

A CIP catalogue record for this book is available from
the British Library.

Printed and bound in China

10 9 8 7 6 5 4 3 2 1

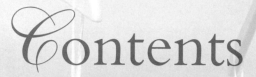

Contents

introduction

CONGRATULATIONS! YOU ARE EMBARKING ON AN EXCITING JOURNEY AND WE WANT TO HELP YOU MAKE YOUR WEDDING DAY A MOST MEMORABLE AND BEAUTIFUL ONE. WITH SO MUCH TO THINK ABOUT AND SO MUCH INFORMATION AVAILABLE, OUR AIM IS TO GUIDE YOU TOWARDS THE RIGHT CHOICE OF DRESS TO WEAR FOR *YOU*, AS WELL AS THROUGH A WHOLE HOST OF OTHER DECISIONS YOU WILL NEED TO MAKE.

colour me beautiful

colour me beautiful Europe has now been established for over 25 years and is the leader in the image consulting industry. With hundreds of consultants Europe-wide, thousands of women (and men) have 'had their colours done' and attended style consultations as well. Finding the colours and styles of clothes that really suit them has helped to develop an image with which they are comfortable and confident, and this has spilled over into their social and professional lives. Our consultants have a wealth of knowledge and experience to share with clients that will ensure the end result is a happy one, which will help them achieve their best whatever the situation.

your big day

Experts are available to help you with wedding etiquette, the type of ceremony you might choose and even the vows you can make. This book focuses on how you can look your very best on your wedding day. It will help you to decide what you and your bridal party should wear, as you will be the centre of everyone's attention. This is *your* day and by understanding yourself and what suits you, you will be able to make your own decisions about what you want to wear and do on your special day. This book is not intended to be prescriptive, as every bride will have her individual personality and her own thoughts about her ideal bridal gown.

You may have dreamt about your wedding day and what you want (and don't want) to wear, although sometimes dreams are simply not realistic. However, this book will show you how to make those dreams as much of a reality as possible, by helping you focus on those things that will make you a truly beautiful bride, completely confident and comfortable in what you are wearing. In the chapters that follow, we will show you:

- The right colours for your complexion.
- The right styles of dress for your body shape.
- How to co-ordinate your look with make-up, hairstyling and accessories that suit your face shape, scale and proportions. Remember that your partner is marrying you, not someone he fails to recognize on the day.
- How to ensure your bridal party co-ordinates with you.
- And finally, how to make your wedding day simply the best.

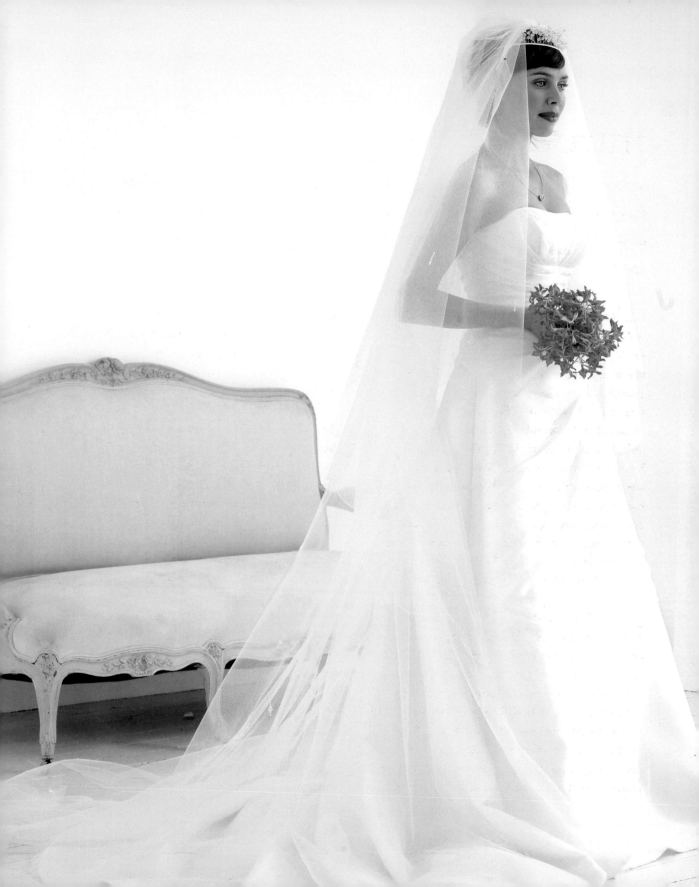

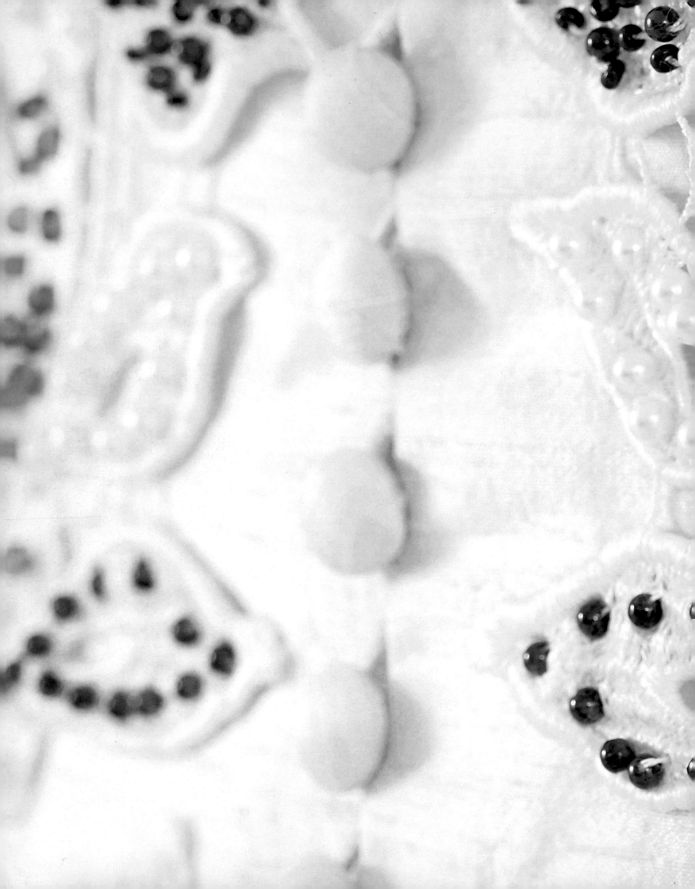

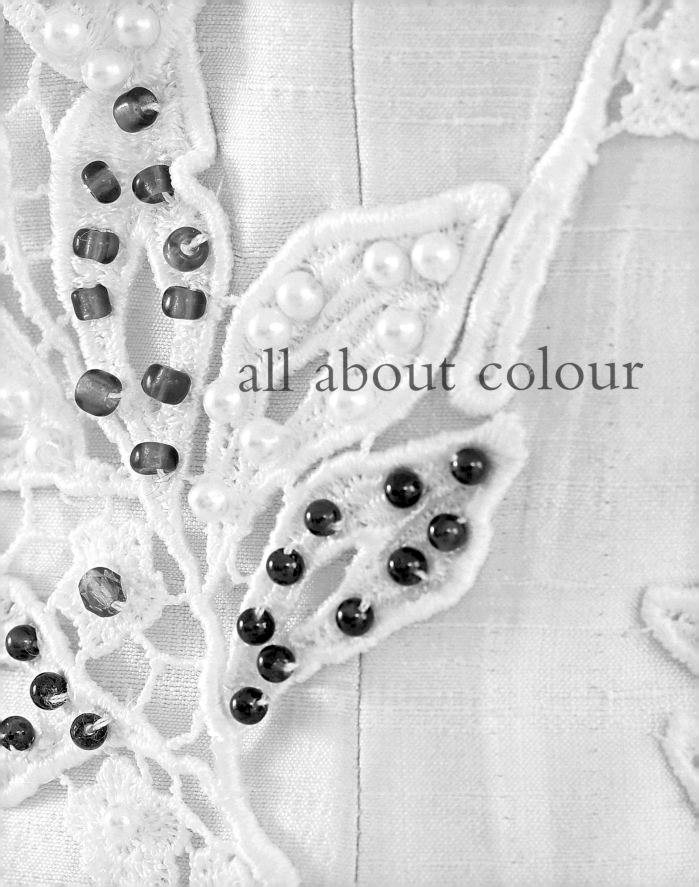

all about colour

considering colour

IN THE WESTERN WORLD, TRADITIONALLY BRIDES WEAR A VIRGINAL PURE WHITE. OVER THE YEARS, HOWEVER, CONVENTIONS HAVE CHANGED. THE AVERAGE AGE OF A BRIDE IS NOW 31 YEARS 6 MONTHS, AND THE NATURE OF MANY WEDDINGS HAS BEEN TRANSFORMED TO ALLOW A MORE FLEXIBLE CHOICE OF COLOURS AND STYLES. IN SOME CULTURES, COLOURFUL WEDDING DRESSES ARE THE NORM, BUT YOU STILL NEED TO ENSURE THAT THE ONE YOU CHOOSE IS THE RIGHT SHADE FOR YOU.

the importance of colour

Many brides will still choose to wear a 'white' dress. However, at **colour me beautiful** we know that there are many shades of white, cream and ivory. So, it is not just a matter of choosing a 'white' dress, but a 'white' that is right for your colouring. This will depend on your skin tone, eye and hair colour.

Whatever colour you wear near your face will reflect upwards on to it. If the colour is in harmony and balance with your natural colouring, you will look healthier and more radiant. If the colour is wrong, it can create shadows, dark circles around your eyes and even give you an uneven complexion, which you may then need to cover with heavier make-up.

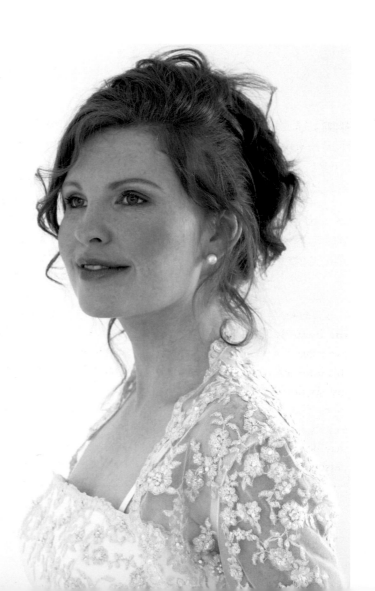

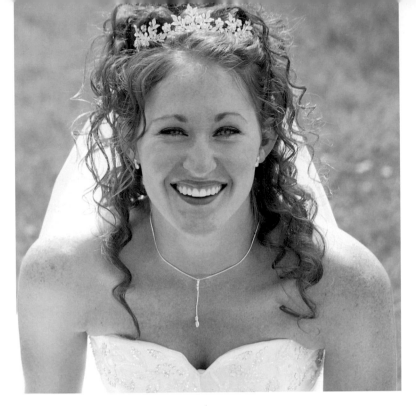

ABOVE *Here we see a bride with warm colouring wearing pure white, which is hard and harsh against her skin tone.*

LEFT *A warm cream-toned wedding dress complements the creamy skin tones of this warm bride.*

Over many years, **colour me beautiful** has developed an extensive colour system, but for this book we have chosen to use just six dominant colouring types. If you find you do not fit exactly into one of these, you may benefit from a detailed personal analysis from a professional consultant.

what is colour?

All colours are made up of three elements:

Depth (light to dark) In other words, how much white there is in a colour – lack of white in a colour deepens its shade and tone.

Undertone (warm or cool) This denotes how much yellow or blue there is in a colour – for more warmth, add yellow; to cool it down, add blue.

Clarity (clear to soft) Clear colours are vibrant and intense, soft colours muted and dusty. Over the following pages you will be able to identify which of the six dominant **colour me beautiful** colouring types you

are: Light, Deep, Warm, Cool, Clear or Soft. You can then use this knowledge to help you select a colour for your wedding dress, as well as those to use as accents for flowers, trims, jewellery and even shoes.

changing colours

Before you establish your colouring, you will need to decide what you want to do with your hair colour (see Tips for the day, on pages 12–17) as this many change your overall appearance. You may even be considering tinted contact lenses, which will also affect your overall appearance. However, be aware that drastic changes may not always work successfully and look natural.

ALTERNATIVE ADVICE

The advice we give on colour applies not only to a traditional wedding dress but also to any alternative outfit you may choose to wear (see pages 68–71). Remember to take a look at bridesmaids' dresses, too, as many of these would make a beautiful wedding dress and may be available in just the colour you want.

light

CHOOSING A WEDDING DRESS IS EASY FOR A BRIDE WITH LIGHT COLOURING. YOUR DELICATE COLOURING WILL BE PERFECTLY BALANCED AND COMPLEMENTED BY ALL SHADES OF WHITE AND CREAM. IF YOU CHOOSE TO USE COLOUR, YOU SHOULD STICK TO LIGHT AND PASTEL SHADES NEAR YOUR FACE.

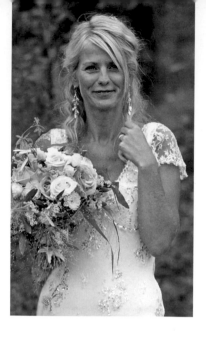

do you have...

- Naturally blonde hair with light eyebrows and lashes?
- Pale, light-coloured eyes?
- Delicate porcelain skin?

the light bride

As your overall look is light and delicate, you are going to look wonderful in all the traditional whites, ivories and creams. Pastels and light colours will also work well. You do not want to be overwhelmed by strong colouring, worn by either yourself or any of the wedding party who might be standing near you. The groom can also lighten his look, even if he is wearing a dark suit.

ABOVE *Ulrika Jonsson has typical light colouring; the soft white colour and delicate fabric of her dress balances with her colouring.*

TIPS FOR THE DAY

- If you want to enhance your hair colour, golden or ash highlights are your best options.
- Your skin tone is delicate, so don't hide it under a fake or real tan.

ACCENT COLOURS

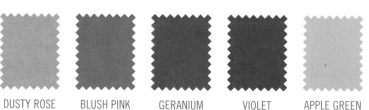

DUSTY ROSE   BLUSH PINK   GERANIUM   VIOLET   APPLE GREEN   PRIMROSE   LIGHT AQUA   SKY BLUE

deep

AS A DEEP BRIDE YOU WILL NEED TO THINK THROUGH YOUR COLOUR OPTIONS CAREFULLY TO ENSURE THAT YOU MAKE THE MOST OF YOUR FABULOUS LOOK. CHOOSING THE RIGHT LIGHT SHADE FOR YOU IS VERY IMPORTANT – HAVE FUN TEAMING IT WITH COLOURFUL ACCESSORIES AND MAKE-UP.

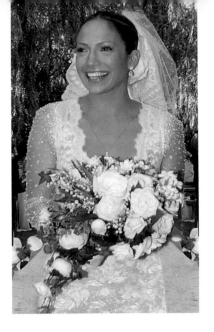

do you have...

- Dark hair?
- Dark eyes?
- Porcelain to dark skin?

the deep bride

On your wedding day you want to look stunning, and if you choose to wear a light-coloured dress you will need to balance it with rich tones in your make-up and accent colours. Your natural colouring will always be best in darker, stronger colours. By being creative and bringing more colour into your look, perhaps with trims or accessories, you will be able to create a dramatic look.

ABOVE *Jennifer Lopez has stunning dark eyes and beautiful dark hair; the low neckline of her dress works well with her colouring.*

TIPS FOR THE DAY

- Don't be tempted to highlight your hair – just keep it in good condition to make it shine.
- Make sure your foundation matches your skin tone perfectly to avoid a mask-like appearance.

ACCENT COLOURS

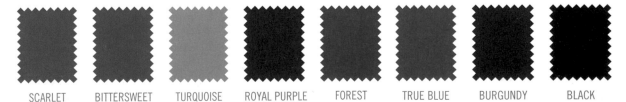

SCARLET   BITTERSWEET   TURQUOISE   ROYAL PURPLE   FOREST   TRUE BLUE   BURGUNDY   BLACK

warm

WARM BRIDES OFTEN HAVE VERY PALE PORCELAIN SKIN WHICH IS BEST
COMPLEMENTED WITH IVORY OR CREAM SHADES. IF FRECKLES ARE
PRESENT, DON'T TRY TO HIDE THEM; TOGETHER WITH THE RED TONES
IN YOUR HAIR THEY WILL BALANCE BEAUTIFULLY WITH COLOURS THAT
HAVE A YELLOW UNDERTONE.

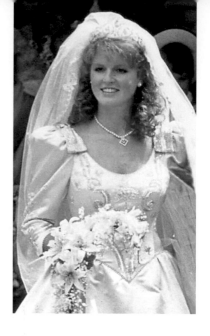

do you have...

- Any shade of red hair, from auburn to strawberry blonde?
- Brown, hazel, green or blue eyes?
- Golden or freckled skin?

the warm bride

Your wonderful warm colouring will be enhanced by all the fantastic ivories, creams and golden shades. If you choose to wear a pure white dress, the addition of texture, embroidery or lace will soften the look of the fabric to balance your skin tone. Golden jewellery will be your best choice, and your make-up colours will need to be yellow-based to co-ordinate with your overall look.

ABOVE *Sarah Ferguson wore a beautifully embellished cream dress, decorated with pearls, and had yellow flowers in her bouquet.*

TIPS FOR THE DAY

- Enhancing the colour of your hair with gold tones will add to your overall golden look.
- If you have freckles anywhere, don't hide them – they are part of who you are.

ACCENT COLOURS

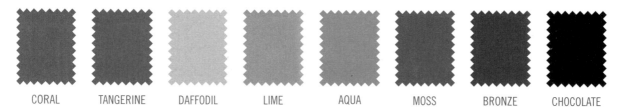

| CORAL | TANGERINE | DAFFODIL | LIME | AQUA | MOSS | BRONZE | CHOCOLATE |

cool

A BRIDE WITH COOL COLOURING WILL LOOK GOOD IN PURE WHITE AND ALL
SHADES OF IVORY. OTHER COLOURS NEED TO HAVE A COOL OR BLUE TONE
TO THEM. IF YOU ARE A COOL BRIDE YOU SHOULD MAKE THE MOST OF
YOUR BEAUTIFUL EYES WITH SHADES OF MAKE-UP THAT COMPLEMENT
RATHER THAN DISTRACT.

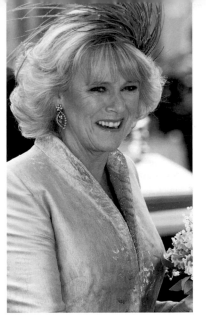

do you have...
- Ash tones or grey hair?
- Blue or grey eyes?
- Rosy skin tone?

the cool bride
With your rosy skin tone you can balance your look with magnificent whites. The creamy yellows are best avoided, but you have the choice of all the icy shades including hints of lavender as well as pinks, blues and mints. By keeping your make-up colours cool-toned, you will ensure a flawless look. Think silver, platinum and the biggest diamond he can afford!

ABOVE *The Duchess of Cornwall chose to wear a silvery-grey wedding dress that made the most of her cool colouring.*

TIPS FOR THE DAY
- Don't try to hide any grey hair – just enhance it with ash-toned tints or highlights.
- Although your make-up colours should remain cool, avoid bright blue eye shadow if you have blue eyes.

ACCENT COLOURS

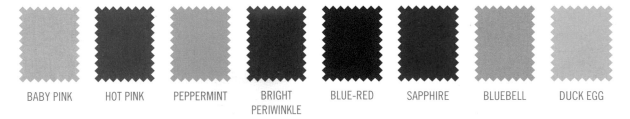

| BABY PINK | HOT PINK | PEPPERMINT | BRIGHT PERIWINKLE | BLUE-RED | SAPPHIRE | BLUEBELL | DUCK EGG |

clear

IF YOU HAVE CLEAR COLOURING THEN THE CONTRAST BETWEEN YOUR HAIR COLOUR, SKIN TONE AND EYE COLOUR NEEDS TO BE COMPLEMENTED WITH COLOURS THAT HAVE IMPACT. SO IF YOU CHOOSE TO WEAR ANY SHADE OF WHITE OR CREAM, BALANCE IT WITH BRIGHTLY COLOURED FLOWERS OR ACCESSORIES.

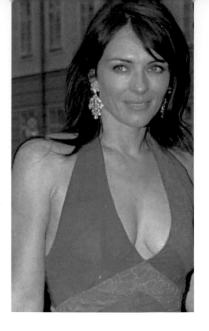

do you have...

- Dark hair?
- Bright blue, green or topaz eyes?
- Pale porcelain skin?

the clear bride

Your striking appearance is best balanced with clear, bright tones. If you choose to wear white or ivory, a sheen on the fabric will add to its clarity. Your hair should give the light-against-dark contrast that is typical of your colouring, while accent colours will do the same against a pale dress.

ABOVE *Liz Hurley chose to wear a bright pink dress to balance with her dark hair, bright eyes and stunning clear look.*

TIPS FOR THE DAY

- Keep to lowlights if you want to enhance your hair colour.
- If you need to wear glasses, make sure you have non-reflective lenses so that your eye make-up colours show through.

ACCENT COLOURS

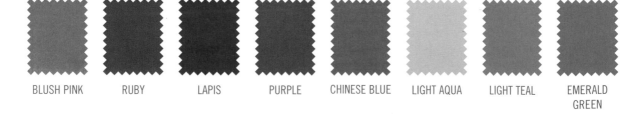

| BLUSH PINK | RUBY | LAPIS | PURPLE | CHINESE BLUE | LIGHT AQUA | LIGHT TEAL | EMERALD GREEN |

soft

YOUR MUTED EYE COLOURING TOGETHER WITH THE BLENDED TONES IN YOUR HAIR MEANS THAT YOU HAVE A CHOICE OF MANY COLOURS THAT WILL LOOK STUNNING ON YOU. SOFT WHITES AND CREAMS WILL BE GREAT FOR A TRADITIONAL LOOK AND TAUPES AND BEIGES ARE FANTASTIC FOR SOMETHING A LITTLE DIFFERENT.

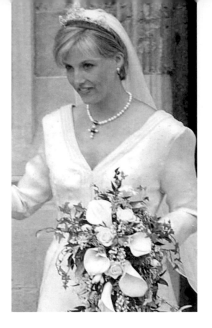

do you have...

- Mousy hair, often highlighted?
- Blended, muted eye tone?
- Neutral skin tone?

the soft bride

The fabulous softness of your look needs to be balanced with gentle tonal colours such as soft whites, ivories and champagne. Your accent colours should be more tonal than high contrast. Fabric with texture will often help to achieve a softer look even if the colour is brighter. You will benefit from your bridal party wearing colours that do not clash or contrast with your own look.

ABOVE *The Countess of Wessex enhanced the soft white of her dress with a stunning pearl necklace and silk chiffon veil.*

TIPS FOR THE DAY

- Your best look is to keep highlighting your hair.
- Matt, textured jewellery and pearls will look fantastic on you.

ACCENT COLOURS

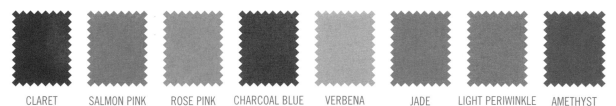

| CLARET | SALMON PINK | ROSE PINK | CHARCOAL BLUE | VERBENA | JADE | LIGHT PERIWINKLE | AMETHYST |

looking good in whites

WHITE IS TRADITIONALLY ASSOCIATED WITH BRIDAL GOWNS. IT COMES IN MANY DIFFERENT SHADES, AND YOU NEED TO MAKE SURE THAT IF YOU GO FOR A REAL WHITE WEDDING DRESS YOU CHOOSE THE VERY BEST WHITE FOR YOU. KNOWING YOUR DOMINANT COLOURING WILL HELP YOU SELECT THE APPROPRIATE SHADE.

which white should you wear?

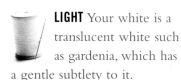 **LIGHT** Your white is a translucent white such as gardenia, which has a gentle subtlety to it.
Fabric Select as sheer a fabric as you can take to balance with your scale: are you petite, average or grand?

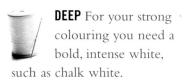 **DEEP** For your strong colouring you need a bold, intense white, such as chalk white.
Fabric The strength of the colour will be enhanced by heavier fabrics.

 WARM The choice of white for you needs a little thought. Balance the warm tones of your colouring with jasmine white, which includes a hint of yellow.
Fabric The use of texture as in a shantung silk will soften the clarity of the white.

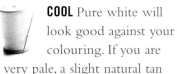 **COOL** Pure white will look good against your colouring. If you are very pale, a slight natural tan will enhance the white.
Fabric Pure white lace gives you the option of softening the 'hard' quality of this colour.

 CLEAR The stunning clarity of orchid white will provide you with a backdrop for a colourful and stunning bouquet.
Fabric Make sure that whatever fabric you choose shines.

 SOFT Your soft white is the gentlest white of all. Its tone can often be achieved by selecting texture in the fabric.
Fabric Matt fabrics will absorb the light and therefore soften the colour.

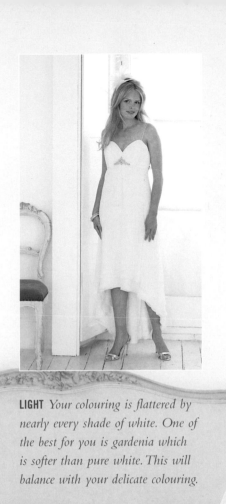

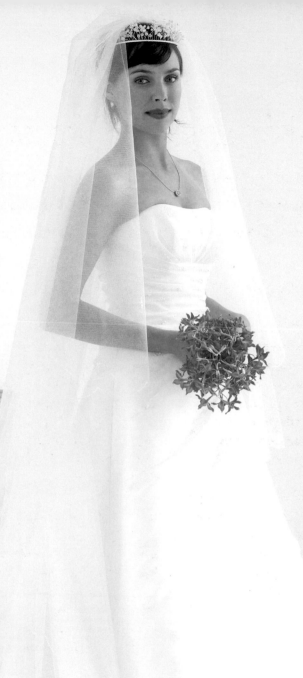

LIGHT *Your colouring is flattered by nearly every shade of white. One of the best for you is gardenia which is softer than pure white. This will balance with your delicate colouring.*

CLEAR *With your contrasting colouring your choice of white needs to be one which has clarity to it. Orchid white is the best option for you; you then have the opportunity of using contrasting accessories to balance your look.*

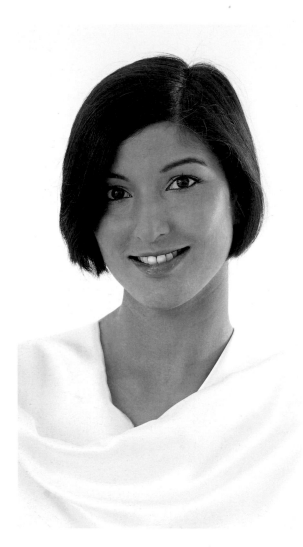

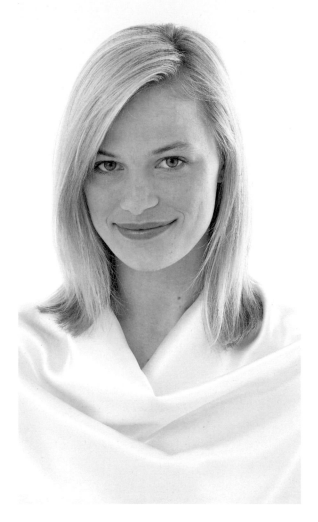

Deep

Chalk white is a deep rich white and will look great in a textured fabric which will intensify the colour. Don't be afraid of some bold coloured flowers in your bouquet, they will offset wonderfully against your chalk white dress.

Cool

Your best white is a pure white that has absolutely no yellow tones in it whatsoever. If you think that this colour might be a little harsh, think about having it in a soft satin or silk, or with an overlay of lace.

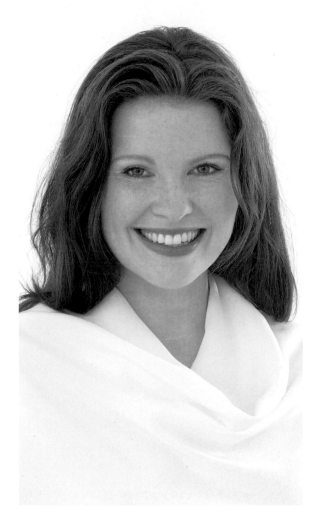

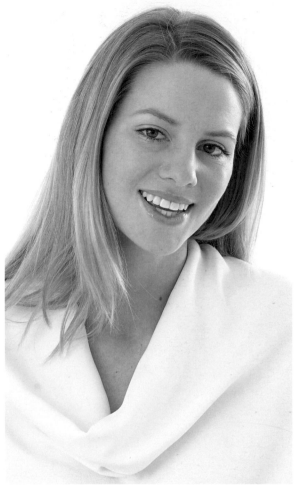

Warm

Your best white is jasmine white with its warm yellow undertones. Make sure that you complement it with make-up colours that are warm-based and link the look with some yellow-toned flowers in your bouquet.

Soft

Soft white is the very best white for your soft muted tones. This white has the clarity taken away from it; often this can be achieved with the correct choice of fabric. Any decorations on the dress should complement and blend with the colour of the dress.

looking good in creams

CREAM WILL SUIT MOST PEOPLE BUT, DEPENDING ON YOUR NATURAL COLOURING, YOU WILL NEED TO ADAPT THE SHADE TO MAKE SURE YOU LOOK A MILLION DOLLARS. THERE ARE MANY TONES TO CHOOSE FROM AND THE TYPE OF FABRIC CAN HAVE A POWERFUL EFFECT ON THE APPEARANCE OF THE COLOUR: THE SAME CREAM SHADE WILL LOOK QUITE DIFFERENT IN A DUCHESS SATIN TO THE WAY IT APPEARS IN A SILK CRÊPE, FOR EXAMPLE. FOR MORE DETAIL ON FABRICS, SEE PAGES 44–45.

which cream should you wear?

 LIGHT The very palest shade of cream, such as ivory, will be best for you as anything too dark might overwhelm your delicate fair colouring.
Fabric You can choose both light-reflecting and matt fabrics.

 WARM Most creams are just made for you and your beautiful warm and golden colouring.
Fabric If you want to add embellishment to your dress, think pearls, gold thread and ribbons and trims.

 CLEAR Your cream will be the brightest you can find, such as champagne, to contrast with the brightness of your eyes and the strength of your hair colour.
Fabric Select fabrics that have a natural sheen or are embellished with sparkles.

 DEEP You need to wear the deepest shade of cream you can find, such as vanilla. Avoid the palest shades.
Fabric To enhance the colour of the fabric and give it richness, use texture, embellishment or lace.

 COOL Your cream will be one with a hint of cool pink, such as a calamine, to balance with your rosy-toned skin. Avoid creams that are yellow-based.
Fabric Choose embellishments and accessories in silver, grey or bluish tones.

 SOFT Medium shades of cream will look gorgeous on you. Oyster will harmonize well with your muted colouring.
Fabric Matt fabrics are your best choice. You can always add lace over the top of a shiny fabric to create the right effect.

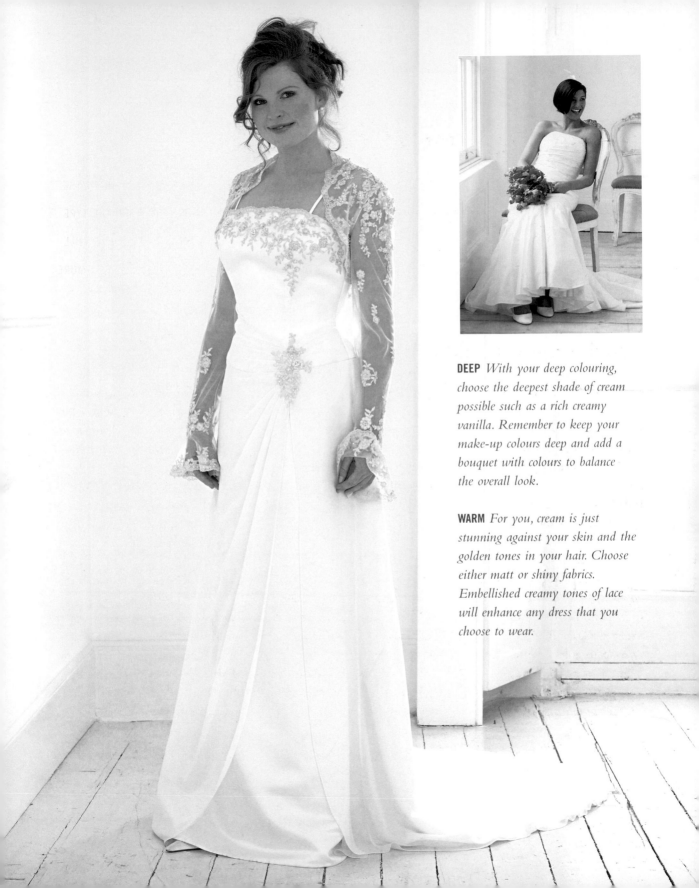

DEEP *With your deep colouring, choose the deepest shade of cream possible such as a rich creamy vanilla. Remember to keep your make-up colours deep and add a bouquet with colours to balance the overall look.*

WARM *For you, cream is just stunning against your skin and the golden tones in your hair. Choose either matt or shiny fabrics. Embellished creamy tones of lace will enhance any dress that you choose to wear.*

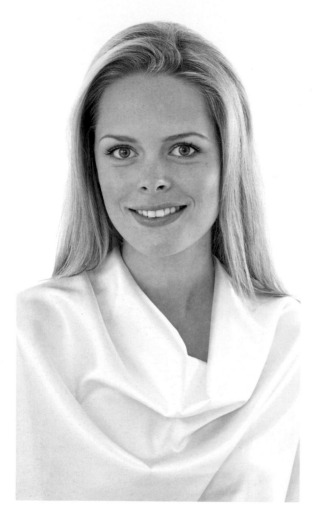

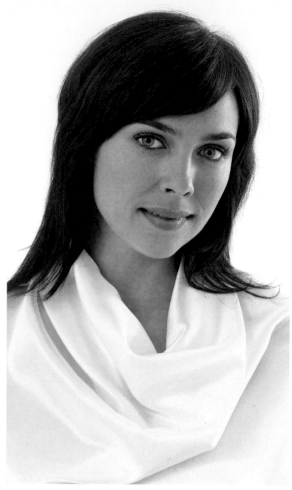

Light

The lightest shades of cream are for you; shades such as ivory balance and enhance the pale colouring of your eyes and porcelain skin – especially if you are going to be wearing a dress that will show off some flesh.

Clear

Champagne, as the name implies, means a cream that is clear and has a slight crispness to it. If your body shape allows, choose a crisp fabric, if not, add some sparkle to the fabric you choose to complement your look.

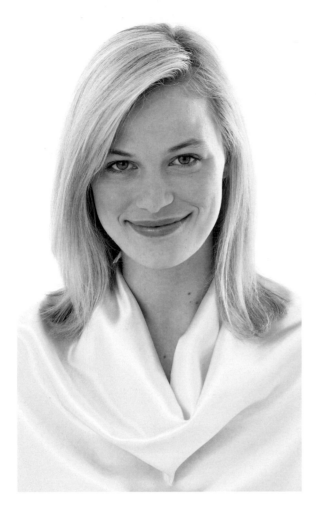

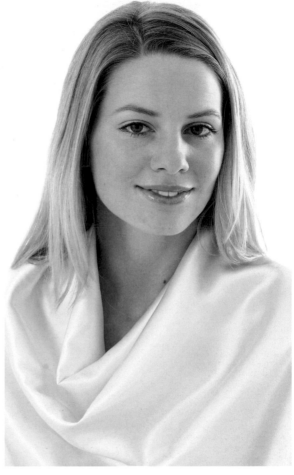

Cool

If you decide to wear cream it needs to have a touch of pink to it, calamine is a wonderful choice. Any pale colour with a hint of rose is perfect for you. Complement the look with pink pearls and silver.

Soft

Think of the inside of an oyster shell and that is the perfect colour for your soft muted colouring. You can go one shade lighter or darker but keep the fabric or finish of the dress as matt as possible.

looking good in beiges

IF YOU THINK A 'WHITE' DRESS IS NOT FOR YOU BUT WANT TO STICK TO A TRADITIONAL BRIDAL COLOUR, CONSIDER ONE OF THE BEAUTIFUL BEIGES THAT ARE AVAILABLE TO SUIT ALL COLOURINGS. BEIGES FORM A PERFECT BACKDROP TO ALL KINDS OF BEADING, EMBROIDERY, LACE OVERLAY AND ACCESSORIES.

which beige should you wear?

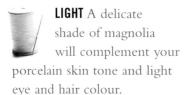 **LIGHT** A delicate shade of magnolia will complement your porcelain skin tone and light eye and hair colour.
Fabric A sheer georgette in your shade of beige will give you the transparent, light shade you need.

 DEEP Your strong colouring can take the deeper shades of beige, such as cocoa.
Fabric A brocade or velvet will provide the richness you need to balance your natural rich and dramatic colouring.

 WARM Antique gold will reflect the warm tones of your hair, skin and eyes beautifully.
Fabric You have the choice of your best shade of beige in most fabrics.

 COOL Your beige needs to be cool – pebble is a perfect example.
Fabric Choose either matt or light-reflecting fabrics.

 CLEAR The brightest of the beiges is taupe, which makes a perfect base for contrasting accents.
Fabric Go for a light-reflecting fabric with a smooth surface.

 SOFT You can choose from a wide selection of beiges, but medium shades such as stone are best.
Fabric Use texture in your fabric to create a tonal look.

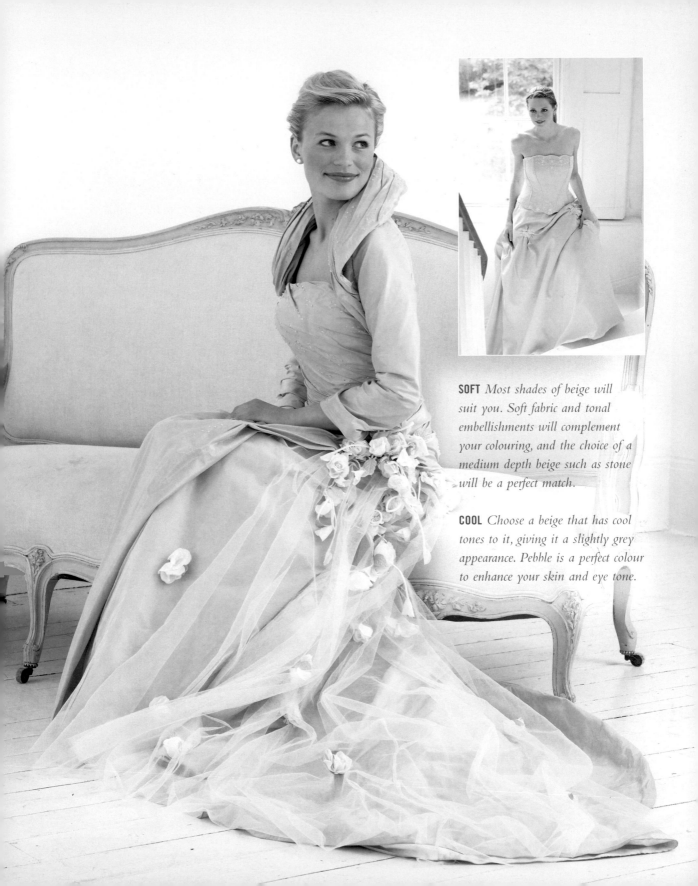

SOFT *Most shades of beige will suit you. Soft fabric and tonal embellishments will complement your colouring, and the choice of a medium depth beige such as stone will be a perfect match.*

COOL *Choose a beige that has cool tones to it, giving it a slightly grey appearance. Pebble is a perfect colour to enhance your skin and eye tone.*

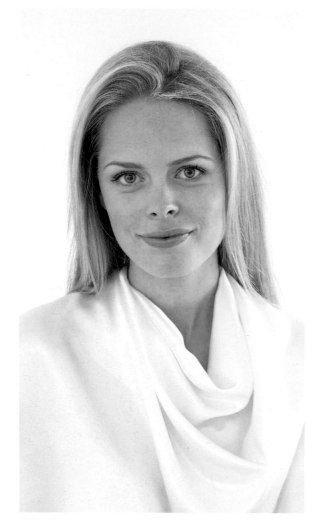

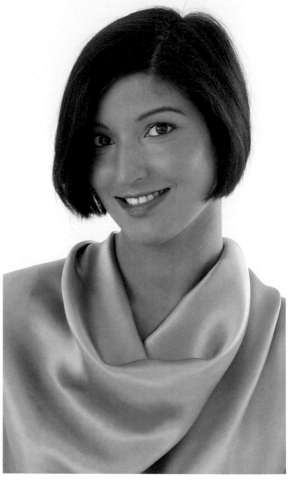

Light

Magnolia is the lightest shade of beige available, and is the perfect colour for the delicate tones of someone with light colouring. Depth can be added in the form of embellishments in slightly stronger shades if you wish.

Deep

The choice of cocoa as your beige will give you the depth and strength of colour that you need to complement your colouring. Rich dramatic colours for your eye shadow will work well with a less dramatic lip colour.

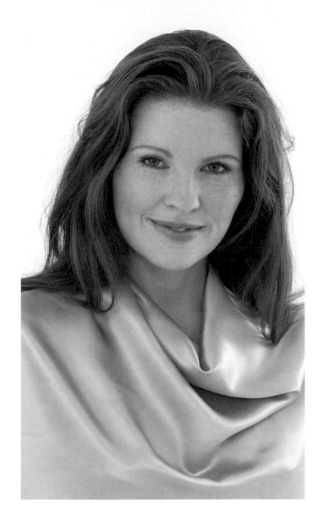

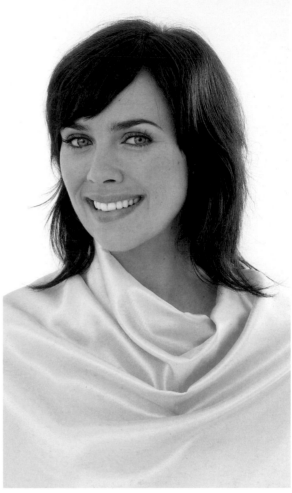

Warm

The perfect beige for you is antique gold which is available in many different fabrics whether shiny or matt. This is a stunning colour for you to wear and is suitable for all types of wedding dress.

Clear

Taupe is a bright shade of beige, so if you are looking for something different for your wedding dress you may choose to wear this, with some added details to complement your clear colouring and bright eyes.

pastel greens

TRADITIONALLY, GREEN WAS NOT CONSIDERED A COLOUR A BRIDE WOULD CHOOSE TO WEAR. HOWEVER, IN TODAY'S ENVIRONMENTALLY AWARE SOCIETY GREEN HAS BECOME INCREASINGLY FASHIONABLE AND POPULAR IN WOMEN'S WEAR. PASTEL GREENS WILL GIVE YOUR WEDDING DRESS A MODERN AND INNOVATIVE LOOK.

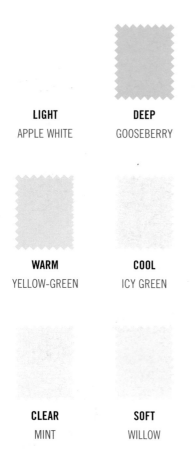

LIGHT
APPLE WHITE

DEEP
GOOSEBERRY

WARM
YELLOW-GREEN

COOL
ICY GREEN

CLEAR
MINT

SOFT
WILLOW

RIGHT *Here our light bride wears a beautiful dress in apple white.*

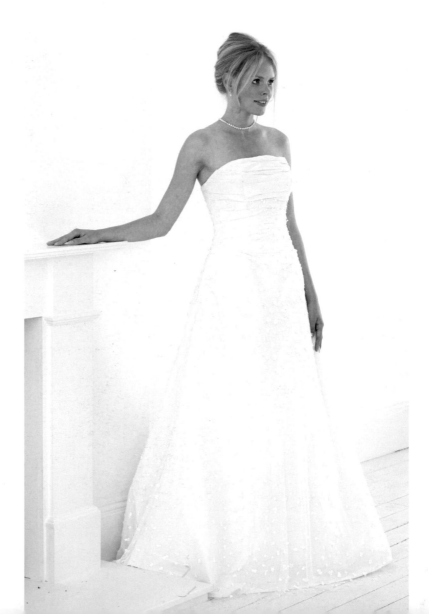

greens

THERE IS SOMETHING CREATIVE AND UNUSUAL ABOUT CHOOSING GREEN FOR YOUR WEDDING OUTFIT. YOUR CHOICE OF SHADE MIGHT BE AFFECTED BY THE TIME OF YEAR: A PINE-GREEN DRESS AT A CHRISTMAS WEDDING WILL SET THE SCENE, WHILE IN SPRING AN APPLE-GREEN GOWN CAN BE FUN AND DIFFERENT.

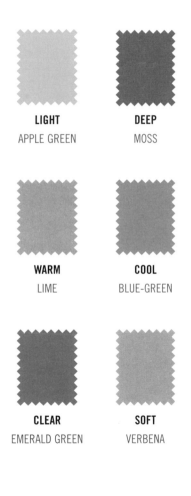

LIGHT
APPLE GREEN

DEEP
MOSS

WARM
LIME

COOL
BLUE-GREEN

CLEAR
EMERALD GREEN

SOFT
VERBENA

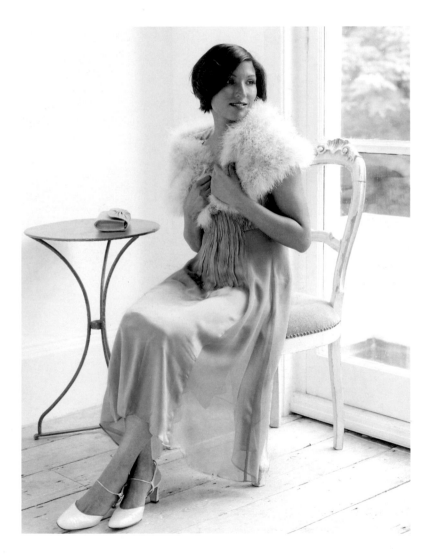

RIGHT *Our deep bride is wearing a vintage-style dress in light moss.*

blues

YOU HAVE A CHOICE OF VARIOUS SHADES OF BLUE DEPENDING ON YOUR DOMINANT COLOURING. YOU CAN LIGHTEN OR DEEPEN YOUR SHADE BY USING THE BLUE AS A BASE FABRIC WITH A SHEER WHITE OR CREAM OVER THE TOP, OR ALTERNATIVELY YOU COULD USE A BLUE GEORGETTE OR LACE OVER WHITE OR CREAM.

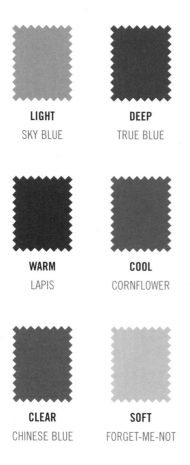

LIGHT
SKY BLUE

DEEP
TRUE BLUE

WARM
LAPIS

COOL
CORNFLOWER

CLEAR
CHINESE BLUE

SOFT
FORGET-ME-NOT

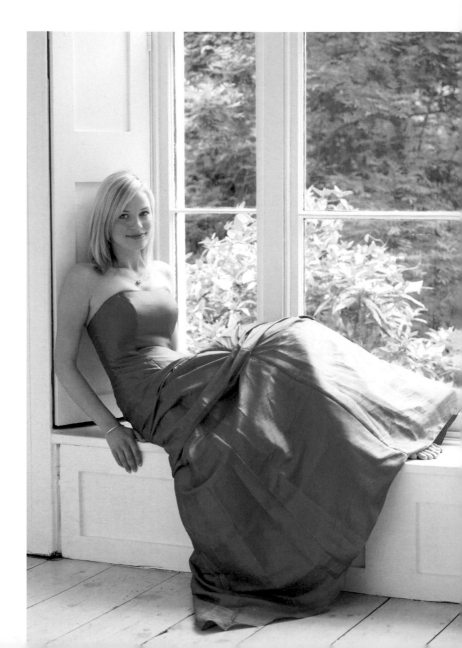

RIGHT *Our cool bride's cornflower dress complements her colouring.*

aquas, teals and light blues

IF YOUR WEDDING IS TAKING PLACE AT THE HEIGHT OF SUMMER OR IN A TROPICAL LOCATION, YOU MIGHT LIKE
TO CHOOSE A BEAUTIFUL AQUA OR TEAL WHICH WILL GIVE A FEELING OF LIGHT AND FRESHNESS TO THE DAY.
LIGHT BLUES ARE FLATTERING AGAINST MOST SKIN TYPES AND A GREAT ALTERNATIVE TO WHITE.

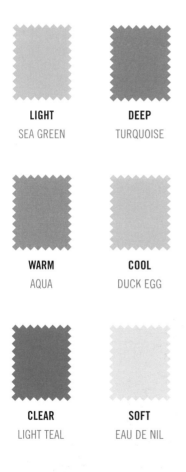

LIGHT
SEA GREEN

DEEP
TURQUOISE

WARM
AQUA

COOL
DUCK EGG

CLEAR
LIGHT TEAL

SOFT
EAU DE NIL

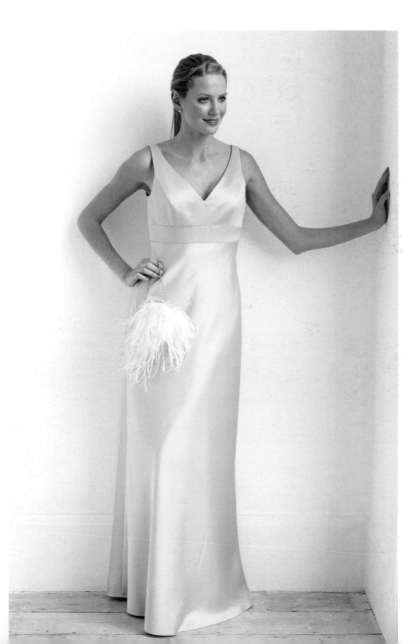

RIGHT *Eau de nil is a perfect choice
for our soft bride.*

pastel pinks

IF YOU HAVE A ROMANTIC AND FEMININE PERSONALITY, YOU MAY CHOOSE TO WEAR PINK ON YOUR WEDDING DAY. THE SHADE YOU CHOOSE FOR YOUR BLUSHER AND LIPSTICK MUST BALANCE AND WORK IN HARMONY WITH YOUR CHOSEN PINK, PARTICULARLY IF YOU ARE WARM OR COOL.

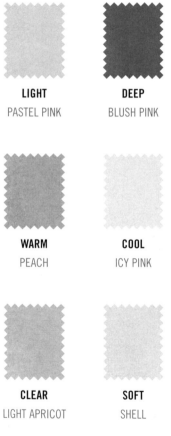

LIGHT
PASTEL PINK

DEEP
BLUSH PINK

WARM
PEACH

COOL
ICY PINK

CLEAR
LIGHT APRICOT

SOFT
SHELL

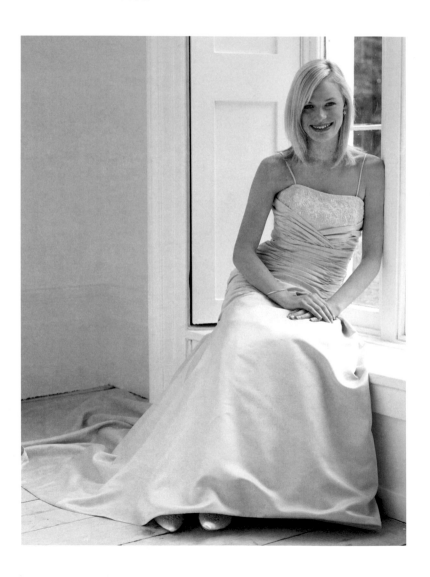

RIGHT *Icy pink balances perfectly with our cool bride.*

reds

TO ADD DRAMA TO YOUR WEDDING DRESS, YOU MAY WANT TO GO FOR RED ON THE DAY. IT CAN BE HEAD TO TOE, OR YOU MAY LIKE TO MAKE YOUR DRESS A TWO-PIECE WITH ONE PART IN RED. IN SOME SOCIETIES, RED IS THE TRADITIONAL WEDDING DRESS COLOUR, SO MAKE SURE IT IS THE RIGHT RED FOR YOU.

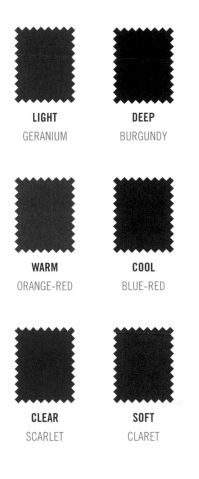

LIGHT
GERANIUM

DEEP
BURGUNDY

WARM
ORANGE-RED

COOL
BLUE-RED

CLEAR
SCARLET

SOFT
CLARET

RIGHT *Burgundy is a stunning match for our deep bride.*

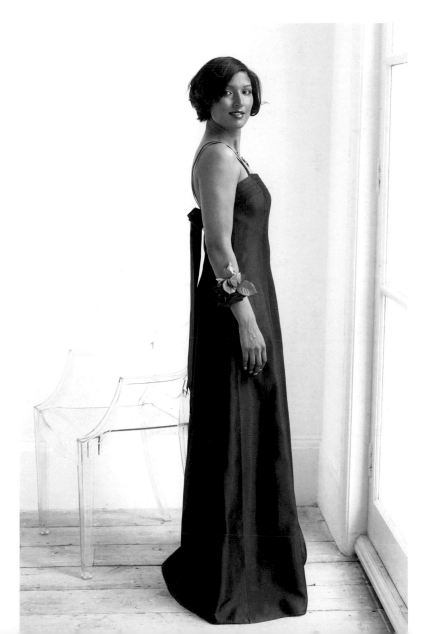

purples

THERE IS NOTHING MORE STUNNING THAN A PURPLE OR BLUE GOWN AT AN EVENING WEDDING. THE DARKER COLOURS ARE VERY FLATTERING AND SLIMMING, WHILE THE SOFTER SHADES WILL HAVE A CALMING AND RELAXING EFFECT ON THE BRIDE AND HER PARTY.

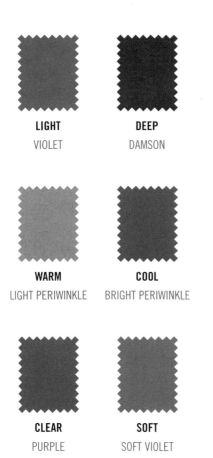

LIGHT
VIOLET

DEEP
DAMSON

WARM
LIGHT PERIWINKLE

COOL
BRIGHT PERIWINKLE

CLEAR
PURPLE

SOFT
SOFT VIOLET

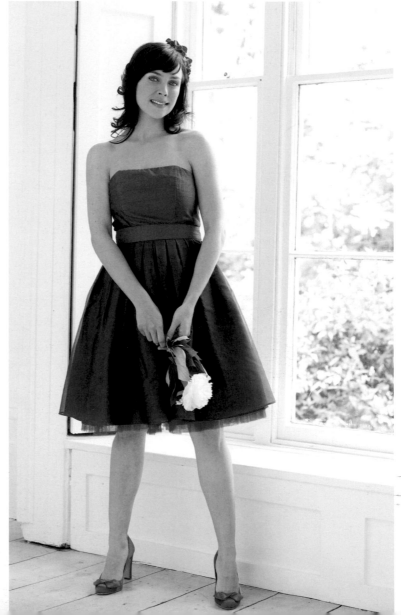

RIGHT *Our clear bride looks amazing in purple and cyclamen pink.*

metallics and blacks

IF YOU REALLY WANT A WEDDING WITH A DIFFERENCE, THEN CHOOSING METALLICS AND/OR SHADES OF BLACK WILL GIVE YOU THE DESIRED EFFECT. ONLY THOSE WITH DEEP COLOURING CAN WEAR BLACK FROM HEAD TO TOE; OTHER COLOURING TYPES SHOULD ONLY USE IT AS A TRIM.

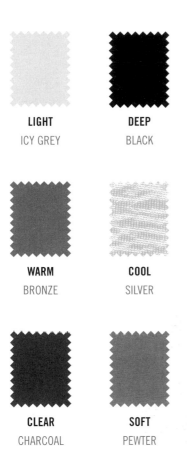

LIGHT
ICY GREY

DEEP
BLACK

WARM
BRONZE

COOL
SILVER

CLEAR
CHARCOAL

SOFT
PEWTER

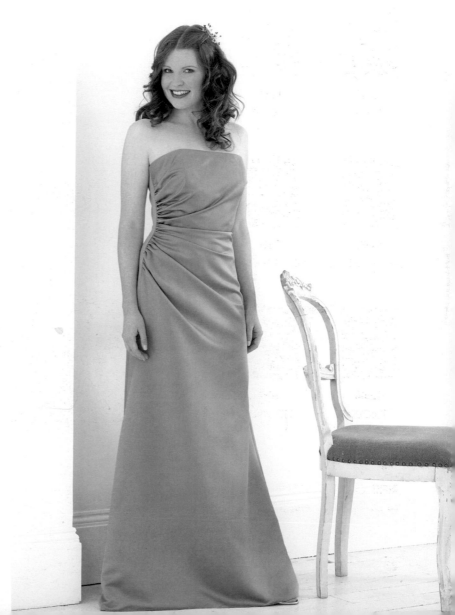

RIGHT *Our warm bride just glows in a bronze wedding dress.*

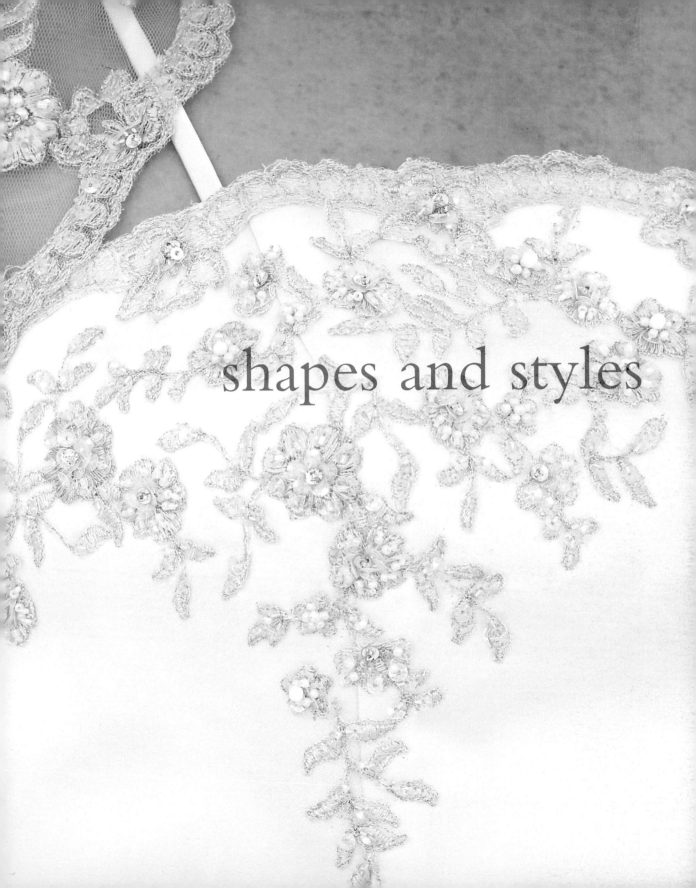

shapes and styles

making it your own

YOU WILL ALREADY KNOW YOUR LIKES AND DISLIKES WHEN CHOOSING CLOTHES. YOU MAY PREFER GARMENTS WITH SIMPLE LINES, OR WOULD RATHER CHOOSE SOMETHING MORE DETAILED AND PRETTY. FOR YOUR WEDDING, YOUR DRESS SHOULD REFLECT YOUR PERSONAL STYLE TO ENSURE THAT YOU FEEL COMFORTABLE WEARING IT ALL DAY. WHATEVER YOUR PREFERENCES, YOU CAN ACHIEVE THE 'WOW' FACTOR WHETHER YOU CHOOSE TO PURCHASE A DRESS OR HAVE IT MADE.

FASHION SENSE

To be that beautiful, confident bride you will need to consider the time of year, the venue, the type of wedding and your own personal preferences. Remember: this is probably not the time to be a victim of high fashion and fads. Your wedding pictures will be brought out on many occasions for years to come, so don't let a crazy fashion fad take over the day.

creative

You will want something completely different from anyone else, perhaps breaking the traditional rules. Choose whatever you like, in colour and/or style. Accessories and embellishments will help you achieve your individual look. Think vintage, ethnic and alternative outfits, one single bloom rather than a bouquet, and a memorable hat or a stunning headdress.

dramatic

There will be nothing understated about your dress or the whole event. Go for it: the bolder, more dramatic will be your way to express your personality on the day. Think about bright colours, lavish accessories or embellishments.

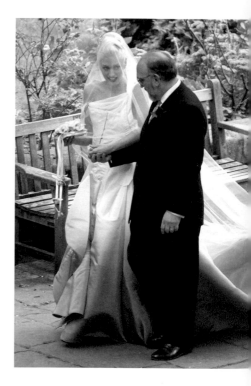

ABOVE *Gwen Stefani's traditional style dress in soft white was dramatised with the shot of deep pink around the skirt and train.*

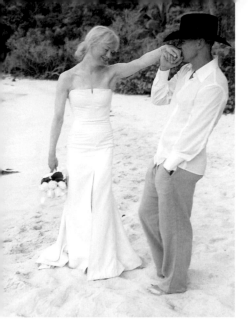

ABOVE *A simple shift dresign was chosen by Renée Zellweger for her relaxed beach wedding.*

romantic

The theme here is pretty, feminine and romantic. You will go for whites and pastel shades, and your dress will have embellishment galore. Enjoy all the pampering and fuss leading up to your wedding. The more romantic styles of wedding dress will be your favourites, and even if you have a rectangle body shape (see pages 46–47), make that shift dress pretty.

classic

Your wedding will be understated but traditional. You do not want a lot of fuss and feel comfortable in a simple dress shape, such as an A-line. However, this is the one occasion when you can break the mould and go for something a little more daring. Add a stunning train, some embellishment on the back of your dress or wear a family heirloom, if available.

natural

You will want to shy away from anything too pretty as you do not do 'special dress'. However, it is your wedding day and it is expected of you to look bridal. The less fitted the dress, the more comfortable you will feel, and there are some stunningly beautiful designs in empire, shift and bias-cut dresses. Choose the one that best suits your body shape (see pages 46–47). You may also like to consider a white trouser suit or a two-piece (jacket plus long skirt) teamed with ballet pumps.

city chic

Your preferred style will be a gown with simple lines, but in a luxurious fabric or using a little embellishment to make it special. You will take time and care in choosing your accessories to show off your fabulous dress. You will keep your bouquet simple, and the whole effect will be one of elegant understatement.

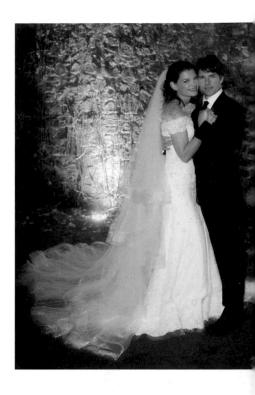

ABOVE *An abundance of frills, flounces and bows adorned Katie Holmes's dream dress.*

HIRING

Whatever style of outfit you go for, look at the possibilities of hiring your dream outfit for your big day. Just make sure you still follow the guidelines in this book.

basic dress shapes

THE BASIC STYLES OF WEDDING DRESS HAVE BARELY CHANGED OVER DECADES. THERE WILL BE FASHIONABLE INFLUENCES AS FAR AS NECKLINES AND FULLNESS OF THE SKIRTS ARE CONCERNED, BUT FUNDAMENTALLY THE SHAPES REMAIN THE SAME. YOU NEED TO IDENTIFY WHICH SHAPE MEETS YOUR ASPIRATIONS WHILE MAKING SURE IT WORKS FOR YOUR BODY SHAPE AND WEDDING STYLE.

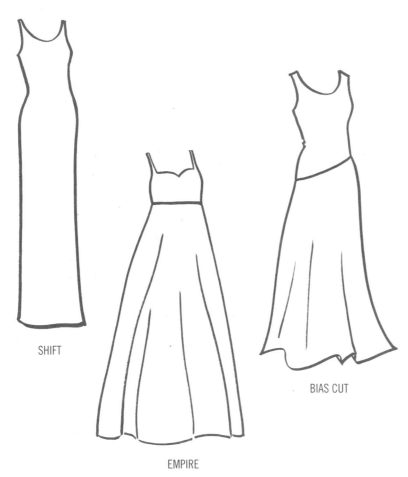

SHIFT

EMPIRE

BIAS CUT

shift

This is basically a simple, straight dress with straight darts that will skim the body. It is ideally suited to stiffer fabrics. The dress can be long or short, and with or without sleeves. It is suitable for all types of wedding. Because of its simplicity, a shift can easily be enhanced with beading, embroidery and lace. If wished, the train can be incorporated into the dress. You may want to consider a slit in the skirt, which will make walking easier as well as adding length to your legs.

empire

This is another simple line, with high waist emphasis just below the bust. The waist detail can be as narrow as a single seam or as wide as a cummerbund. This is

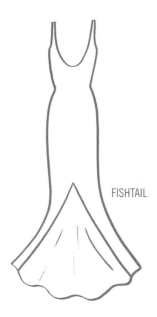

FISHTAIL

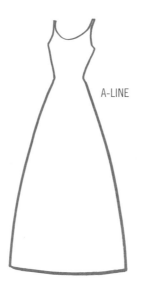

A-LINE

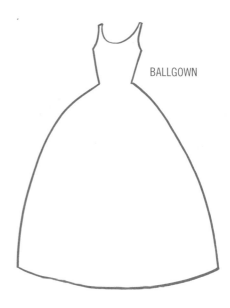

BALLGOWN

a good shape if you are small-busted. The skirt will flare out gently from where the waist seam finishes and its fullness should be determined by your height: the taller you are, the fuller the skirt can be. This is a wonderful style to wear if you are going for comfort first or in a flowing fabric if you are a mother-to-be.

bias cut

The secret of the bias-cut dress lies in the cutting of the fabric. This is done across the grain of the cloth and gives a soft, fluid and feminine look to the finished dress, which will skim the hips gently. It is much more suitable for softer fabrics. If you wish to incorporate a floating, fluid train, this is the ideal style to choose.

fishtail

The fishtail is a variation of the shift, with slightly more waist emphasis and a close-fitting skirt that fans out at the bottom, either all round or just at the back. This really works best on a long style and is ideal for decorating all the way round. It creates a very glamorous look which will give the illusion of longer legs. However, take care where the skirt starts to flare to ensure you can walk easily.

A-line

This dress style is in between the shift and the ballgown. The top is fitted and the skirt flares out as little or as much as you want. This style is ideally suited to a two-piece combination and is therefore the most flexible

for many brides as you can mix fabrics and colours. For extra detail, pleats can be added to the skirt part of the dress if you need to enhance your hips.

ballgown

This is the dress most brides dream about. The bodice is closely fitted and the skirt very full. It is extremely beautiful with its layers upon layers of fabric, petticoats and train, often intricately decorated with beads, pearls and sequins, but it is not always the most practical dress to wear – it is warm in winter but not so good in the summer. If you are petite, keep the skirt volume to a minimum. This style works particularly well if you have long legs or want to disguise full hips or thighs.

fabrics

YOUR WEDDING DRESS IS ONE OF THE MOST EXPENSIVE DRESSES YOU WILL EVER BUY. THE FABRIC YOU SELECT WILL PLAY A KEY ROLE IN MAKING THAT DRESS FIT PERFECTLY AND THIS IS THE MAKE OR BREAK OF THE PERFECT WEDDING DRESS. YOU WILL ALSO NEED TO CONSIDER WHAT EMBELLISHMENT, IF ANY, YOU WANT TO ADD TO THE FABRIC.

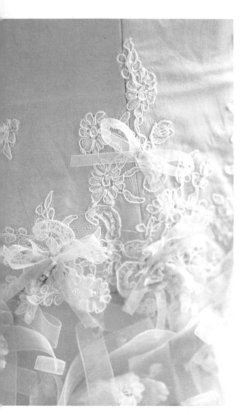

ABOVE *Lace and ribbons can both be used to add detail.*

fabric factors

When you are looking at fabrics, there are three elements to consider:

Weight This is determined by the number of fibres spun into the thread of the yarn. The higher the number, the heavier the fabric. Lightweight fabrics have a fluid feel and will drape more easily.

Texture This is created by the weaving process and will give a smooth or raised finish. Some textures produce a matt finish, others shiny; some weaving processes, such as that used for damask, give a fabric matt and shine together.

Fluidity This depends on the type of yarn and the weaving process. Some fabrics, such as georgette, are loosely woven, which produces an easy draping characteristic. Tightly woven fabrics, like satin, drape less easily and feel crisp.

selecting a fabric

The chart opposite provides a guide to the three elements of weight, texture and fluidity for a range of fabrics and will help you make an informed choice. You may have your heart set on a luxury yarn such as silk, but do not reject silk mixes out of hand as these are far less prone to creasing and it may be easier to incorporate embellishments.

lace

Most laces have their origins in earlier centuries in continental Europe. Lace is often used to enhance a plain-textured fabric or to add details to the dress. There are many different styles and weights of lace available, most originating from traditional and regional designs. When choosing lace, you will need to consider both weight, texture and the type of fabric it's being worn with.

Alençon Needlepoint lace with a raised motif on sheer net, outlined with heavier silk cording, known as gimp.

Chantilly Delicate floral and ribboned design in heavy thread on a mesh background. Edges are scalloped.

Guipure Heavy, very textured lace with a raised design, connected by threads.

Ribbon Not strictly a lace but ribbons sewn into patterns on various weights of net.

Spanish Flat lace usually with a rose design.

Venetian Heavy lace with a raised, floral or geometric design on an open background.

EMBELLISHMENTS

Embellishments are added to a fabric to emphasize the style or to add details to a simple design. They can also enrich the fabric, giving it texture and individuality. Embellishments can be as simple as a few pearls or sequins added to the edge of a sleeve or as complex as an all-over pattern. Silk flowers and bows can add a touch of colour that may link to your flowers and bridesmaids' or even groom's outfits. Just make sure any embellishment does not draw attention to an area of your body you would rather not show off!

FABRIC	WEIGHT*	TEXTURE	FLUIDITY
brocade	heavy	raised	crisp
chiffon	light	minimal	very fluid
damask	heavy	raised	crisp
duchess satin	variable	minimal	variable
dupion	variable	slight	variable
georgette	light	minimal	fluid
moiré	variable	subtle	variable
organza	light	minimal	crisp
shantung silk	variable	slubbed	variable
silk crêpe	variable	crinkled or grained	variable
taffeta	light	minimal	crisp
velvet	heavy	plush	medium

*Some fabrics are available in variable weights, which will affect their fluidity.
In these cases, the lighter the fabric, the more fluid it will be.

your body shape

YOUR SIZE DOES NOT DETERMINE YOUR BODY SHAPE. WHATEVER SIZE YOU ARE, UNDERSTANDING YOUR BODY SHAPE WILL ENABLE YOU TO FINE TUNE THE CHOICE OF DRESS STYLES THAT WILL COMPLEMENT YOU BEST. YOU MAY FIND YOU FALL BETWEEN TWO SHAPES, IN WHICH CASE YOU WILL NEED TO COMPARE WHICH DRESSES HAVE THE HIGHER STAR RATING IN BOTH SECTIONS (SEE PAGES 48–59). THE GREATER THE NUMBER OF STARS, THE BETTER THE DRESS STYLE IS FOR YOU.

neat hourglass

Your bust is well defined and you have soft curves to your hips, bottom and tummy. You generally have little difficulty in getting clothes to fit, so most styles will suit you as long as your proportions are balanced.

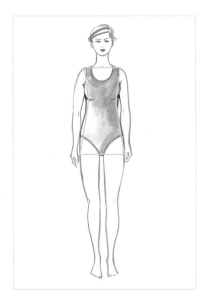

full hourglass

You have a full bust, a well-defined waist, full hips and possibly a curvy bottom. If you get a good fit on the hips you will often find the waist of skirts and trousers is too large. Close-fitting designs are your best bet.

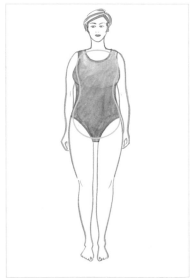

triangle

Your bust may be minimal or full, and your shoulders probably narrow and sloping. You will have difficulty finding a shift dress that fits properly. A dress with a full skirt will work well, as will separates.

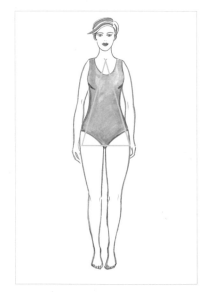

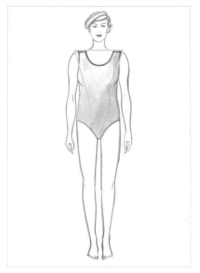

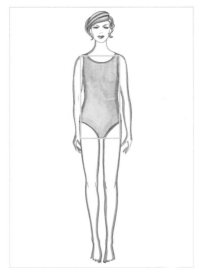

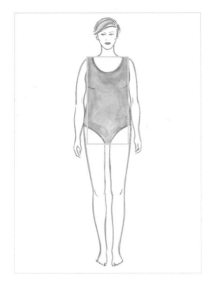

inverted triangle

You may have a minimal or defined waist. Dresses that show off your shoulders are great for your shape. Straight-line styles work well on you, but avoid frills and flounces. You have the perfect shape to add details to your hips and bottom, if you wish.

column

Your appearance is lean and long as you have a minimal bust, just a little shaping around your waist, and flat hips and bottom. You need to consider a dress that really enhances your body shape. A boned bodice and a fuller skirt will work well for you.

rectangle

You may be full or flat chested and your ribcage seems to go straight down to your waist. Your hips and bottom are flat, and you may carry a little weight around your middle. Straight styles are best for you, so look for a dress that gives the illusion of a waist.

SCALE AND PROPORTIONS

When selecting a wedding dress, make sure that you take into account your scale (petite, average, grand) and proportions (high waisted, low waisted) as this will affect the suitability of various designs.

• If you are petite then you should keep the details of your look small and delicate.

• If you have a larger-boned structure you will be able to scale up the details and accessories.

• If you are low waisted, a wedding dress style such as empire line, that gives the illusion of longer legs, will be perfect.

• If you are high waisted, try a dress with a dropped waistline.

neat hourglass

MOST DRESS STYLES WILL LOOK STUNNING ON YOU, SO YOU CAN TAKE YOUR PICK TO FIND YOUR DREAM DRESS. HOWEVER, YOU WILL NEED TO TAKE INTO CONSIDERATION YOUR HEIGHT AND WHETHER YOU ARE HIGH OR LOW WAISTED.

★★★★★ EXCELLENT   ★★★★ VERY GOOD   ★★★ GOOD   ★★ NOT GREAT   ★ NOT FOR YOU

BIAS CUT ★★★★★ In soft fabric, this will drape over your figure beautifully and give you a floaty, ethereal look. This dress is best in a fluid and matt fabric.

A-LINE ★★★★★ This is the style that will flatter your balanced body shape and work well whatever your height and proportions. For a straighter silhouette, choose a crisp fabric such as brocade. For a softer line, choose a silk crêpe.

FISHTAIL ★★★★ This is a wonderful dress to show off your figure. It will give you a very feminine and curvy look. If you are not wearing a veil, there will still be interest at the back. Beware if you are petite, as the fishtail can make you look shorter.

EMPIRE ★★★★ This style will help to enhance a small bust. It will also give an illusion of longer legs. You can alter the look of the dress by mixing different fabrics and textures for the top and bottom – say, lace on top and satin below.

BALLGOWN ★★★★ This is a real Cinderella dress if you are average to grand in height. Make sure that the volume of the skirt does not overpower your bone structure. In a crisp fabric, pleating will be better for the skirt; soft fabrics are better gathered.

SHIFT ★★★ This will be a comfortable dress to wear but will not show off your figure. The softer the fabric, the more shape will be seen.

RIGHT *A bias cut dress will hide nothing, so it is the perfect choice for a neat hourglass.*

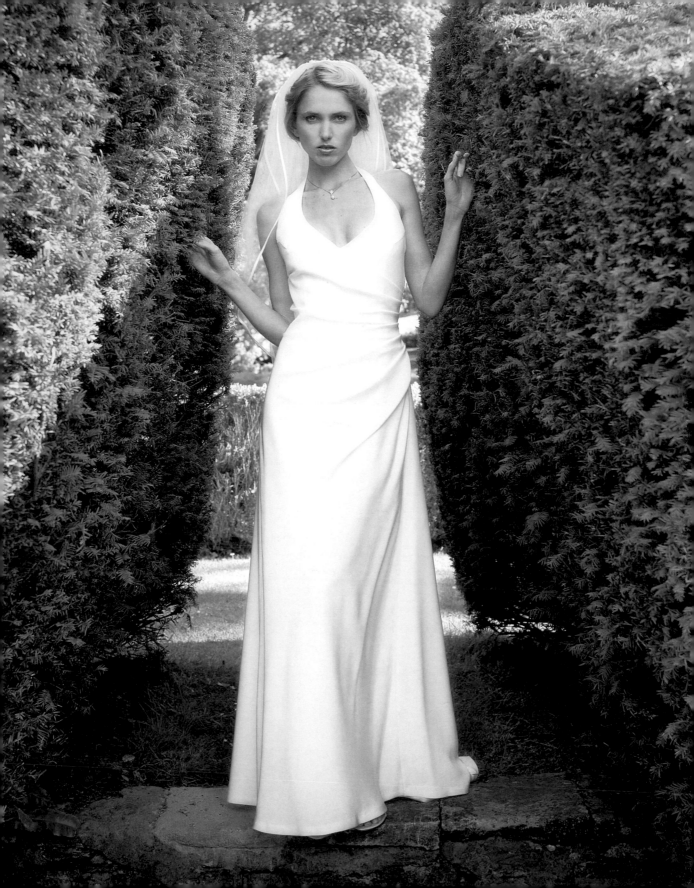

full hourglass

YOUR VOLUPTUOUS FEMININE FIGURE WILL BENEFIT FROM A CLOSE-FITTING DRESS IN SOFT FABRIC. THIS IS A FABULOUS OPPORTUNITY TO SHOW OFF YOUR TINY WAIST, FULL BUST AND CURVY HIPS.

★★★★★ EXCELLENT   ★★★★ VERY GOOD   ★★★ GOOD   ★★ NOT GREAT   ★ NOT FOR YOU

BALLGOWN ★★★★★ The ballgown will emphasize your small waist, and if you want to disguise your hips and bottom this dress is for you. The skirt fabric should be held in soft gathers rather than pleats.

FISHTAIL ★★★★★ Your fishtail dress needs to be created in a soft silk or satin. Beware of gathers over the hips as this will add volume. You will need to balance the depth of the fishtail with your height and leg length.

BIAS CUT ★★★★ This dress is ideal for the average to petite bride. Careful choice of fabric is essential, as it needs to drape over your curves – soft silk crêpe is ideal.

A-LINE ★★★★ This shape is good for you when used as separates. The bodice can be boned to enhance your full bust and the skirt softly flared over your curved hips and bottom.

EMPIRE ★★ The empire shape will accentuate your full bust and should be enhanced with a wide cummerbund just below the waist to show off your lovely curvy figure.

SHIFT ★ The shift dress will work best for you if you add some form of waist definition, such as a half-belt tied at the back, a narrow full belt or a waisted jacket worn over the top. Make sure the fabric of the dress is soft.

RIGHT *A ballgown dress is what dreams are made of and it is perfect for you.*

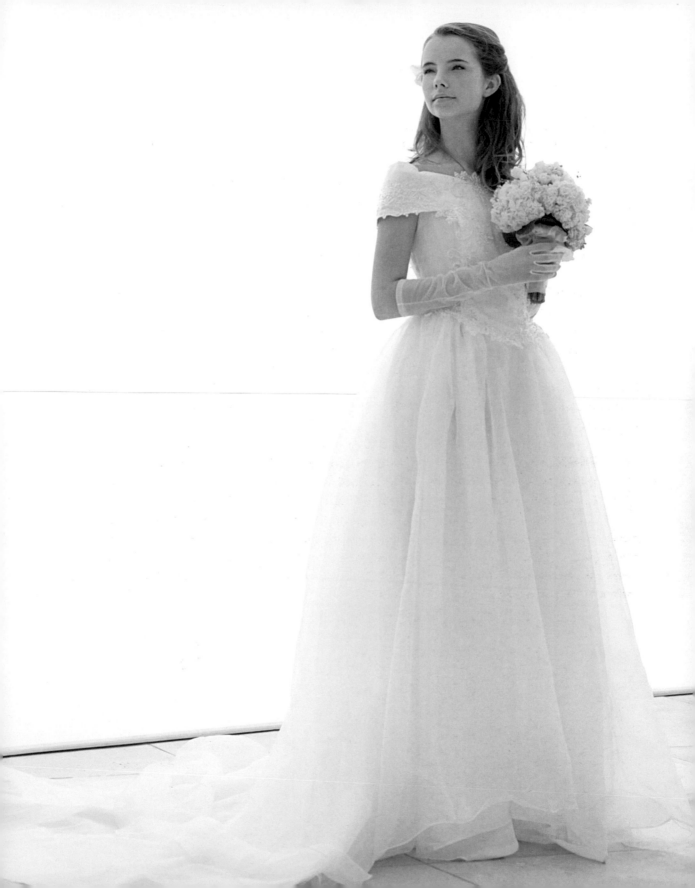

triangle

TO GIVE THE ILLUSION OF YOUR BODY BEING BALANCED, YOU NEED TO BRING ATTENTION AND DETAILS TO THE TOP HALF. THIS CAN BE DONE SUCCESSFULLY WITH FABRICS, LAYERING AND EMBELLISHMENTS.

★★★★★ EXCELLENT ★★★★ VERY GOOD ★★★ GOOD ★★ NOT GREAT ★ NOT FOR YOU

EMPIRE ★★★★★ The empire style of dress lends itself to the addition of all kinds of details to the top half. Because of the loose-fitting skirt, your hips become invisible.

A-LINE ★★★★★ Have fun with the top half of your dress with a bolero, lace or embroidery. Keep the skirt volume down and pleating at the front or back of the skirt.

BALLGOWN ★★★★ Your fairytale dress needs a wide shoulder line to counterbalance the full skirt. Keep the fabric of the skirt simple and fluid.

FISHTAIL ★★ The fishtail dress will not hug your hips. It should look great on you if the detail is actually in the tail, which should start at knee level, thereby balancing the hips.

BIAS CUT ★ This figure-hugging dress needs some interest added to the top and layering if it is to work for you. This could be in the form of a sheer coat or jacket that will float gently over your hips. Shoulder details will draw attention to the top half.

SHIFT ★ To enable this style to fit properly, take the option of making it a two-piece. If you alter the top of a shift dress to fit you, the balance will change and it will not hang properly.

RIGHT *An empire wedding dress style will flatter you as well as giving ease of movement.*

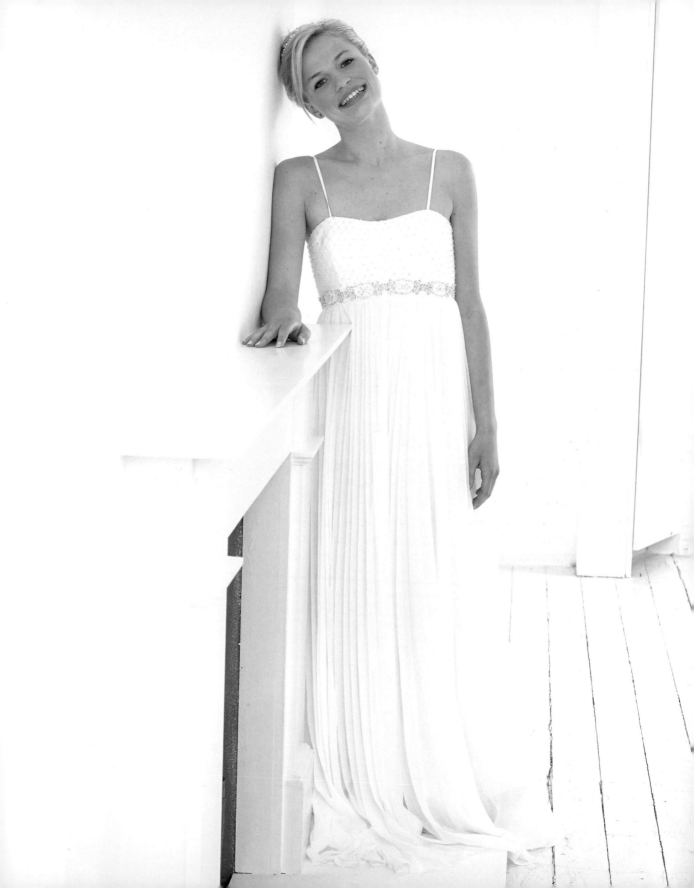

inverted triangle

YOU HAVE FANTASTIC SHOULDERS AND NARROW HIPS. THIS GIVES YOU THE OPPORTUNITY TO BRING ATTENTION TO THE LOWER HALF OF YOUR GOWN WHILE SHOWING OFF YOUR BEAUTIFUL SHOULDERS. YOU WILL FIND CRISPER FABRICS WORK WELL OVER THE STRAIGHT LINES OF YOUR BODY FOR AN UNCLUTTERED LOOK.

★★★★★ EXCELLENT   ★★★★ VERY GOOD   ★★★ GOOD   ★★ NOT GREAT   ★ NOT FOR YOU

FISHTAIL ★★★★★ A strapless style in crisp fabric with gentle ruching over the hips, flaring out at the bottom, will give you an amazing shape.

SHIFT ★★★★★ This slightly waisted dress in crisp fabric will follow the straight lines of your body. Think about adding peplums or exaggerated pleats over the hips for added interest and to balance your shoulder line.

EMPIRE ★★★★ Your choice of empire-style dress should always be in crisp fabric, hanging straight from underneath the bust – no gathers for you. If you have a cummerbund, it should be pleated rather than ruched.

A-LINE ★★★★ Make sure your skirt is flat fronted, with pleats at the side to balance your silhouette. A close-fitting top with minimal embellishment will work well.

BALLGOWN ★★ If you are set on this dress style, again keep the fabric as crisp as possible and avoid gathers and rounded details. The top needs to be straight and fitted with an angled neckline.

BIAS CUT ★ This dress will not hang properly on your figure. However, if this is your dream look, layer it with Venetian lace in geometric designs and patterns.

RIGHT *A fishtail dress will emphasize your figure and create interest below the knees.*

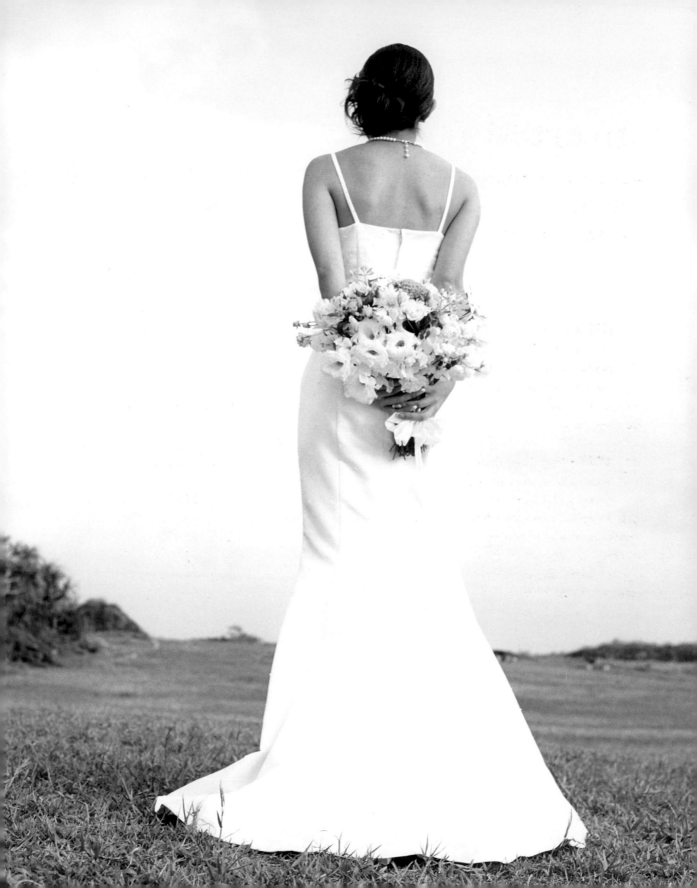

column

YOUR SVELTE FIGURE WILL BE ENHANCED BY USING TEXTURE AND INTERESTING DESIGN FEATURES ON YOUR DRESS. IF YOU ARE ALSO PETITE, MAKE SURE THE WEIGHT OF THE FABRIC DOES NOT OVERWHELM YOUR FINE BONE STRUCTURE.

★★★★★ EXCELLENT   ★★★★ VERY GOOD   ★★★ GOOD   ★★ NOT GREAT   ★ NOT FOR YOU

A-LINE ★★★★★ This dress can be made to enhance your upper body with a boned bodice to give you a fuller bust, which in turn will define your waist. The A-line of the skirt can be achieved with crisp fabrics or using flat pleats.

SHIFT ★★★★ The simple style of this dress will benefit from embellishment, particularly in the bust and hip areas. If you are petite, this style will add height; if you are tall, consider a wide train.

EMPIRE ★★★★ By using textured or patterned fabrics such as brocade or lace, this dress shape will enhance your bust area. A soft, gathered skirt will give you a floaty, feminine look.

FISHTAIL ★★★ You have the perfect body for an Edwardian-style fishtail dress, with a lacy top and a bustle skirt to create detail over your hips and bottom.

BALLGOWN ★★ To make your ballgown work, it will need details above the waist such as sleeves and/or an interesting neckline. If you are at all bony, a beautiful lace covering over the bodice up to the neck will look very elegant.

BIAS CUT ★ The simple elegance of this shape will need to be enhanced by all-over embellishment or layering of the fabric.

RIGHT *A simple A-line dress will be elegant and all the focus will be on you.*

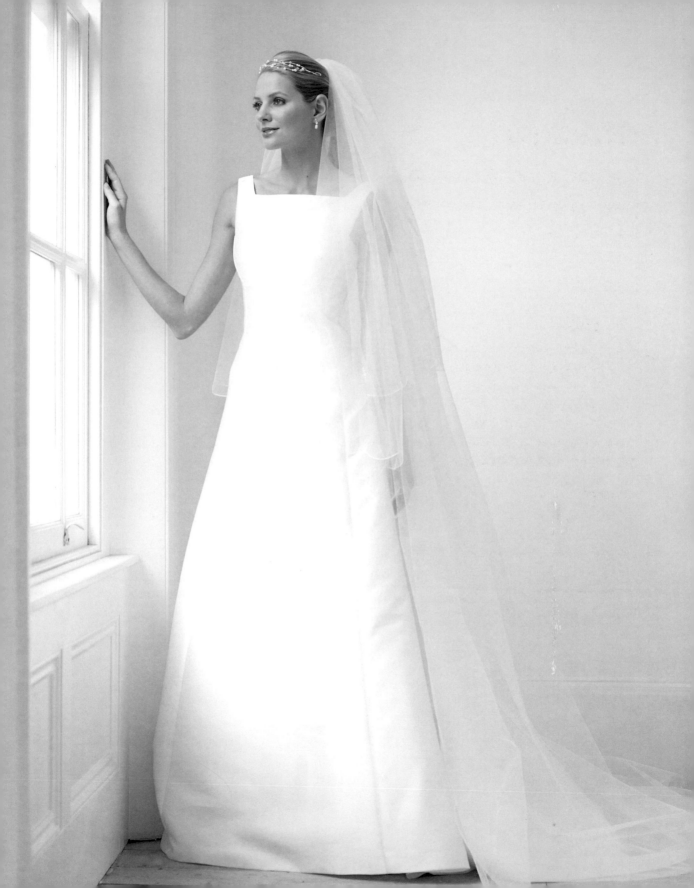

rectangle

THE RIGHT CHOICE OF FABRICS WILL ENSURE THAT YOUR DRESS STYLE COMPLEMENTS YOUR BODY SHAPE. AVOID FINE, CLINGING FABRICS UNLESS YOU USE THEM LAYERED. YOUR BEST OPTION IS A CRISPER, HEAVIER SATIN OR BROCADE. THE SILHOUETTE OF THE DRESS SHOULD BE KEPT SIMPLE, AND MADE SPECIAL BY ADDING EMBELLISHMENTS AND DETAILS.

★★★★★ EXCELLENT   ★★★★ VERY GOOD   ★★★ GOOD   ★★ NOT GREAT   ★ NOT FOR YOU

SHIFT ★★★★★ The straight lines of the shift dress will follow your body shape and make sure you are comfortable all day long. Details such as sleeves, an interesting neck line and a train can make this simple dress the most glamorous one for you.

EMPIRE ★★★★ For a more feminine touch, an empire style wedding dress will enable you to use slightly softer fabrics in the skirt. The seaming under the bust should be kept narrow. Feel free to add details to the back of the dress.

BIAS CUT ★★ The secret to making this dress work for you is to have it in a heavy, matt duchess satin or dupion. This will ensure the dress hangs straight and enhances your figure.

BALLGOWN ★ If this is your choice of dress it needs to be as simple as possible with the least amount of gathering at the waist. A dropped V-shape bodice will ensure that the skirt lies flat over your tummy.

MOTHER-TO-BE

If you are expecting a baby and have lost your waistline, you will be temporarily a fuller-shaped rectangle. In this case, the best dresses for you are the empire and shift styles in soft fabrics only.

FISHTAIL ★★★ Your style of fishtail dress should skim gently over your body with details on the bust and hips. It can be quite tight-fitting on your legs – make sure you have a split in it to enable you to walk.

A-LINE ★★★ The A-line will work for you if the bodice has a dropped waistline. The skirt should lie flat and flare out gently.

RIGHT *A shift dress will look striking with embellishment and details, such as petal sleeves.*

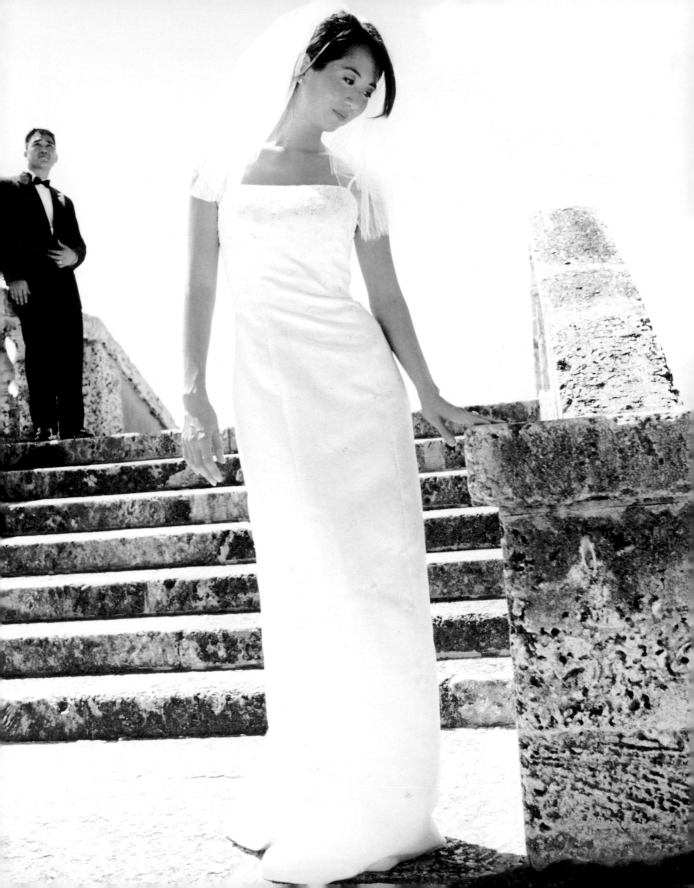

details: bodices and waistlines

THE BODICE IS THE TOP PART OF THE GOWN AND IS OFTEN WHAT MAKES OR BREAKS THE DRESS FOR YOU.
YOU WILL NEED TO CONSIDER THE SHAPE OF THE NECKLINE (SEE PAGES 62–63) AND HOW FITTED THE BODICE
SHOULD BE, PARTICULARLY IF YOU HAVE SELECTED AN EMPIRE, A-LINE, FISHTAIL OR BALLGOWN.

beautiful bodices

The bodice can be simply shaped with seams or darts, as in a bias-cut or shift dress, or elaborate, with boning as in a corset type. Quite often the bodice will be embellished (see page 45). The back is as important as the front and may be one of the most intricate parts of the dress. The bodice must fit perfectly and might need to be refitted at the last minute if you have lost weight, as often the whole structure of the dress hangs from it. If you have an average-sized bust, you can try all the different types of bodice.

perfect waistlines

The shape of the bodice also includes the waistline, which can be positioned at various points depending on proportions.

RIGHT *Remember that many people will see you from the back!*

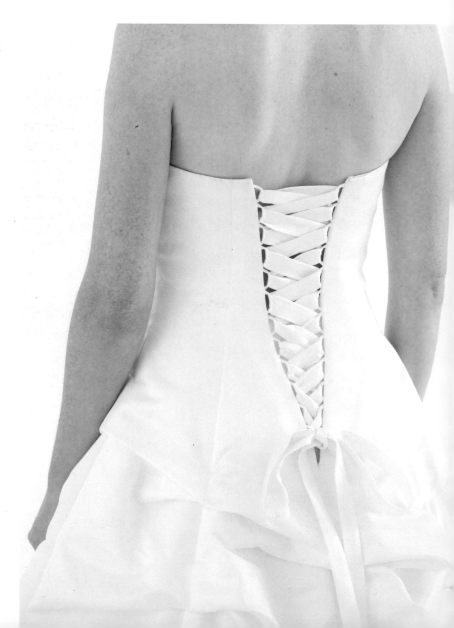

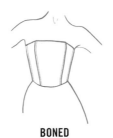

BONED

FULL BUST • SMALL BUST

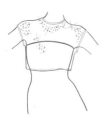

OVERLAY

SMALL BUST

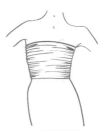

RUCHING

SMALL BUST

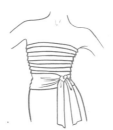

PLEATING

SMALL BUST

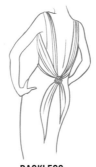

BACKLESS

SMALL BUST

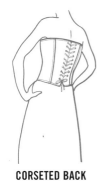

CORSETED BACK

FULL BUST • SMALL BUST

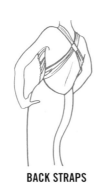

LACING AT BACK

FULL BUST • SMALL BUST

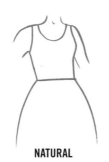

BACK STRAPS

FULL BUST • SMALL BUST

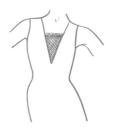

INSERT

SMALL BUST

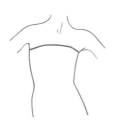

STRAPLESS

SMALL BUST

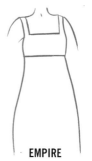

EMPIRE

LOW WAIST • NO WAIST

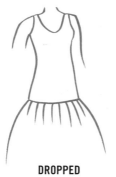

NATURAL

LOW WAIST • HIGH WAIST

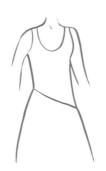

ASYMMETRIC

HIGH WAIST • NO WAIST

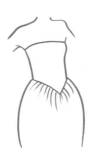

V-SHAPED BASQUE

HIGH WAIST

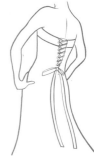

DROPPED

HIGH WAIST • NO WAIST

details: necklines

WHATEVER THE STYLE OF YOUR DRESS, YOU NOW NEED TO THINK ABOUT THE BEST NECKLINES FOR YOU. YOU WILL NEED TO CONSIDER THE LENGTH OF YOUR NECK, ITS WIDTH, YOUR UPPER CHEST, AND HOW COMFORTABLE YOU ARE WITH SHOWING SOME FLESH AND CLEAVAGE.

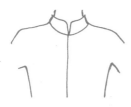

EDWARDIAN/MANDARIN

LONG NECK • THIN NECK
• SMALL BUST

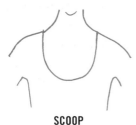

SCOOP

LONG NECK • WIDE NECK •
WIDE, STRAIGHT SHOULDERS
• NARROW, SLOPING SHOULDERS
• FULL BUST • SMALL BUST

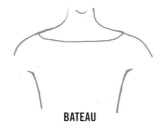

BATEAU

THIN NECK • FULL BUST • SMALL BUST

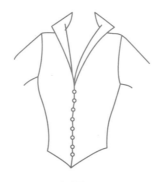

STAND UP

LONG NECK • WIDE NECK • THICK NECK
• WIDE, STRAIGHT SHOULDERS •
NARROW, SLOPING SHOULDERS
• FULL BUST • SMALL BUST

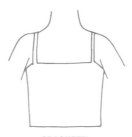

SPAGHETTI

SHORT NECK • WIDE NECK •
WIDE, STRAIGHT SHOULDERS

RIGHT *A sweetheart neckline is enhanced with details below the bust.*

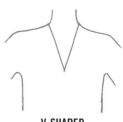

V-SHAPED

SHORT NECK • WIDE NECK
• WIDE, STRAIGHT SHOULDERS
• NARROW, SLOPING SHOULDERS
• FULL BUST

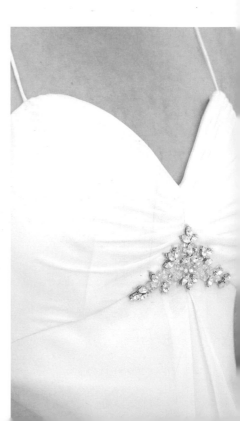

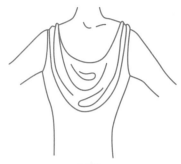

COWL
SHORT NECK • WIDE NECK • THIN NECK
• NARROW, SLOPING SHOULDERS
• FULL BUST • SMALL BUST

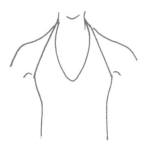

HALTER
WIDE, STRAIGHT SHOULDERS

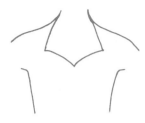

SWEETHEART
LONG NECK • SHORT NECK •
WIDE NECK • THIN NECK
• WIDE, STRAIGHT SHOULDERS •
NARROW, SLOPING SHOULDERS
• FULL BUST • SMALL BUST

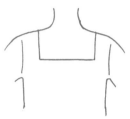

SQUARE
SHORT NECK •
WIDE, STRAIGHT SHOULDERS
• NARROW, SLOPING SHOULDERS

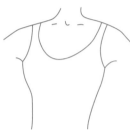

TANK
SHORT NECK • WIDE NECK
• WIDE, STRAIGHT SHOULDERS

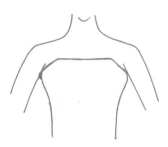

STRAIGHT STRAPLESS
LONG NECK • SHORT NECK
• WIDE NECK • THICK NECK
• WIDE, STRAIGHT SHOULDERS
• SMALL BUST

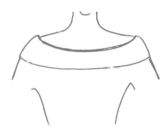

BARDOT
LONG NECK • SHORT NECK • THIN NECK
• NARROW, SLOPING SHOULDERS •
FULL BUST • SMALL BUST

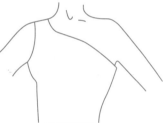

ASYMMETRIC
LONG NECK • THICK NECK •
WIDE, STRAIGHT SHOULDERS
• SMALL BUST

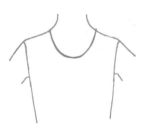

JEWEL
LONG NECK • THIN NECK
• WIDE, STRAIGHT SHOULDERS
• NARROW, SLOPING SHOULDERS •
FULL BUST • SMALL BUST

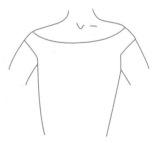

OFF THE SHOULDER
LONG NECK • SHORT NECK • WIDE
NECK • THICK NECK • FULL BUST
• SMALL BUST

details: sleeves

FASHION OR THE TIME OF THE YEAR DICTATE THAT MOST STYLES OF WEDDING GOWN COME WITHOUT SLEEVES. HOWEVER, THIS MAY NOT ALWAYS BE SUITABLE AND YOU SHOULD CONSIDER A RANGE OF FACTORS THAT MAY MEAN YOU WOULD PREFER A DRESS WITH SLEEVES.

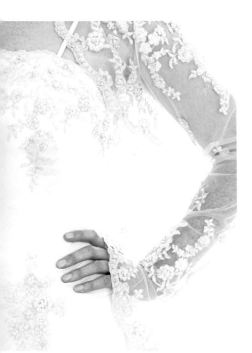

ABOVE *Not everyone has perfect arms, or you might have a winter wedding. Here a beautiful lace shrug is the perfect solution.*

sleeves or sleeveless

Think about the following when making a decision as to whether or not your dress should be sleeveless:

• Type of ceremony, as you may want your arms covered.

• General condition of your arms.

• Length of your arms.

• Size of your bust.

• Fullness, or otherwise, of your upper arms.

If sleeves are simply not available for your chosen style of dress, consider a cover-up in the form of a bolero, jacket, coat or cape (see page 88).

making a choice

There are many types of sleeves suitable for either a dress or a cover-up. The fabric you choose for your sleeves doesn't necessarily have to be the same as that for the main body of the dress. You may want to consider lace, chiffon and other see-through fabrics to give the illusion of a sleeve but without the weight.

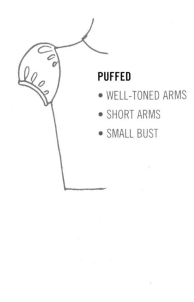

PUFFED
• WELL-TONED ARMS
• SHORT ARMS
• SMALL BUST

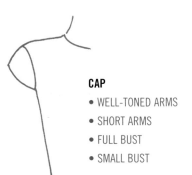

CAP
• WELL-TONED ARMS
• SHORT ARMS
• FULL BUST
• SMALL BUST

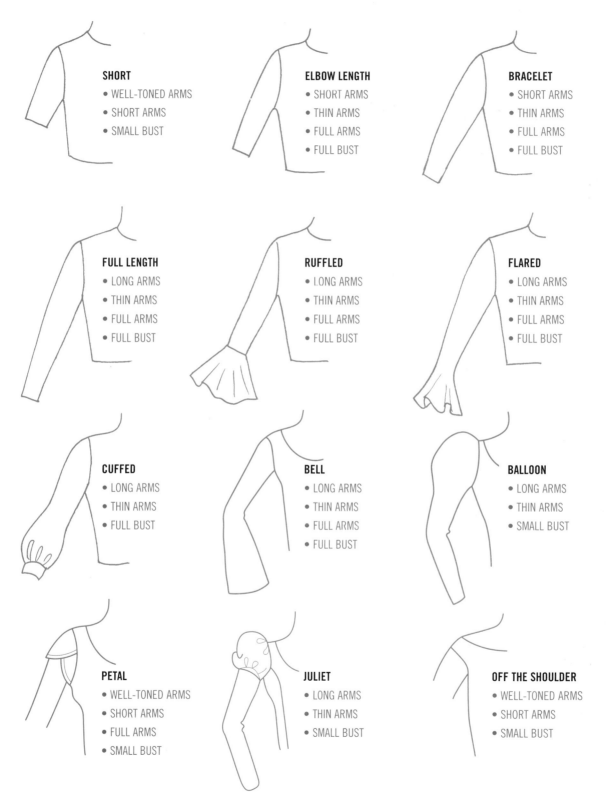

SHORT
- WELL-TONED ARMS
- SHORT ARMS
- SMALL BUST

ELBOW LENGTH
- SHORT ARMS
- THIN ARMS
- FULL ARMS
- FULL BUST

BRACELET
- SHORT ARMS
- THIN ARMS
- FULL ARMS
- FULL BUST

FULL LENGTH
- LONG ARMS
- THIN ARMS
- FULL ARMS
- FULL BUST

RUFFLED
- LONG ARMS
- THIN ARMS
- FULL ARMS
- FULL BUST

FLARED
- LONG ARMS
- THIN ARMS
- FULL ARMS
- FULL BUST

CUFFED
- LONG ARMS
- THIN ARMS
- FULL BUST

BELL
- LONG ARMS
- THIN ARMS
- FULL ARMS
- FULL BUST

BALLOON
- LONG ARMS
- THIN ARMS
- SMALL BUST

PETAL
- WELL-TONED ARMS
- SHORT ARMS
- FULL ARMS
- SMALL BUST

JULIET
- LONG ARMS
- THIN ARMS
- SMALL BUST

OFF THE SHOULDER
- WELL-TONED ARMS
- SHORT ARMS
- SMALL BUST

details: trains

YOU MAY HAVE DREAMT OF HAVING A TRAIN ON YOUR WEDDING DRESS AND NOW IS YOUR CHANCE TO DO IT IN REGAL STYLE. A BEAUTIFUL LONG TRAIN WILL CHANGE THE FEEL OF YOUR DRESS, THE WAY YOU WALK AND THE FORMALITY OF THE OCCASION.

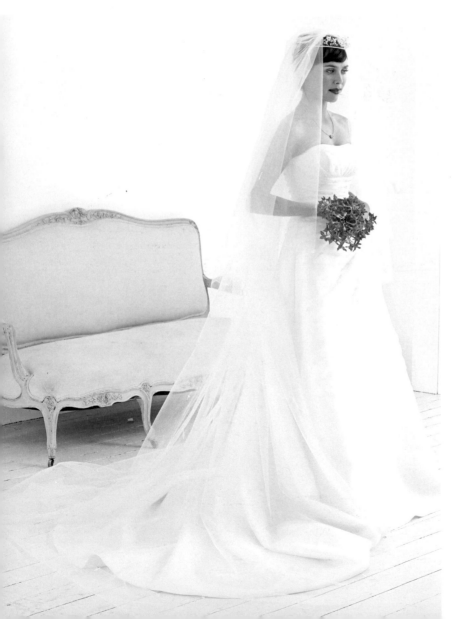

making a choice

The overriding factors in your choice are the shape of your dress and the practicalities of it all. The train will give added weight to your dress and you may even want to consider having it made to be detached when appropriate. An alternative is a train made in a lightweight fabric that will give a more fluid and floaty feel.

PRACTICALITIES

Don't forget that if your train is permanently attached to your dress you will need to think of how you walk, sit and dance with it. There are various ways to help you hold it. These include: a loop you can attach to your wrist, a tape that enables you to ruche up the train, or cleverly positioned hooks and eyes.

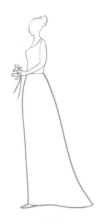

SWEEP

SHIFT • EMPIRE • BIAS CUT • FISHTAIL •
A-LINE • BALLGOWN

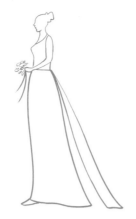

PANEL

SHIFT • EMPIRE • FISHTAIL • A-LINE
• BALLGOWN

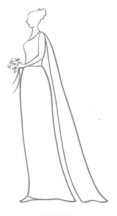

WATTEAU

SHIFT • EMPIRE • A-LINE

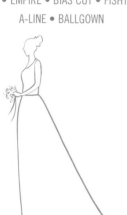

COURT

SHIFT • EMPIRF • BIAS CUT • FISHTAIL
• A-LINE • BALLGOWN

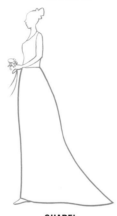

CHAPEL

EMPIRE • BIAS CUT • FISHTAIL • A-LINE
• BALLGOWN

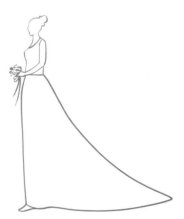

CATHEDRAL

BIAS CUT • FISHTAIL • A-LINE
• BALLGOWN

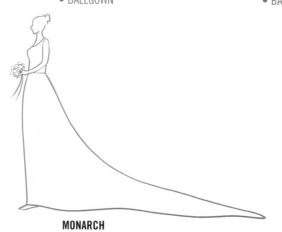

MONARCH

A-LINE • BALLGOWN

LEFT *This beautiful ballgown-style
dress has a full cathedral train as
part of the skirt.*

alternative outfits

YOU MAY DECIDE THAT A FORMAL BRIDAL GOWN IS NOT WHAT YOU WANT TO WEAR AT YOUR WEDDING, OR YOU MAY HAVE DONE THE FORMAL BRIDAL GOWN BEFORE. THERE ARE MANY ELEGANT ALTERNATIVES WHERE YOUR BEST COLOURS AND STYLES CAN COME INTO THEIR OWN.

making a choice

There are several alternative outfits from which to choose:

- Three-piece outfit.
- Evening/cocktail dress.
- Dress and coat.
- Trouser suit.

Aspects you need to consider when choosing what to wear include your personality, the style of the occasion, the likely weather, the venue and what you feel comfortable wearing.

The rules of dressing your body are the same whatever you decide to wear.

jackets and coats

Neat hourglass Most styles will suit you, as long as you choose the right length. If you are petite, a short coat and dress combination will make you appear taller; alternatively, a short jacket and long skirt will achieve the same objective. Also make sure the sleeves stop at the break

of your wrist. If you are grand scale, some definition (belt, pockets, revers) using a contrasting colour or other details will break the length and take the attention where you want it.

Full hourglass Focus on fabrics that have a draping quality. Avoid sharp revers – a soft collar or collarless jacket or coat will work well. Also avoid details (including pockets) over the bust and hips. A jacket with a peplum (a flared ruffle coming from the waist) will look good.

Triangle Consider choosing a patterned jacket or coat over a plain dress or skirt to bring attention to the top half of your body. Interesting embellishments on the jacket can also help to achieve this.

Inverted triangle A constructed jacket with crisp, sharp lines and straight darts will skim your silhouette. Ensure

a jacket finishes at hip level to balance with your shoulders.

Column A slightly waisted jacket or coat with details in the bust and hip areas will give the illusion of a shapely body. Avoid very soft, floaty fabrics.

Rectangle A jacket or coat with some shaping at the waist will work for you. The fuller your shape, the softer the fabric should be. Avoid details on the jacket such as full belts and frills.

skirts

Neat hourglass To ensure your skirt fits properly, you will need a waistband and some darting. Skirts should finish at a point where your leg is narrow – above the knee, on the knee or at the lower calf.

Full hourglass Try a skirt that has some shaping, such as bias cut, flip or panelled. A straight skirt will ride up and may look too small for you.

Triangle Make sure that your skirt does not curve under or grab your fullest part – it needs to hang straight from that point. Avoid too much volume.

Inverted triangle You can choose a skirt with straight-line details such as pleating, panelling or stitching. A skirt with some kick at the bottom will help to balance your shoulders.

Column Consider an A-line skirt that has a slight flare to it. Details and patterns on the skirt will also be good for you.

Rectangle Choose a skirt with no waistband or a drop waist. Straight styles are good, and if the skirt is long a slit will provide a little glamour.

RIGHT *A stylish and detailed suit makes a great alternative to a classic wedding dress.*

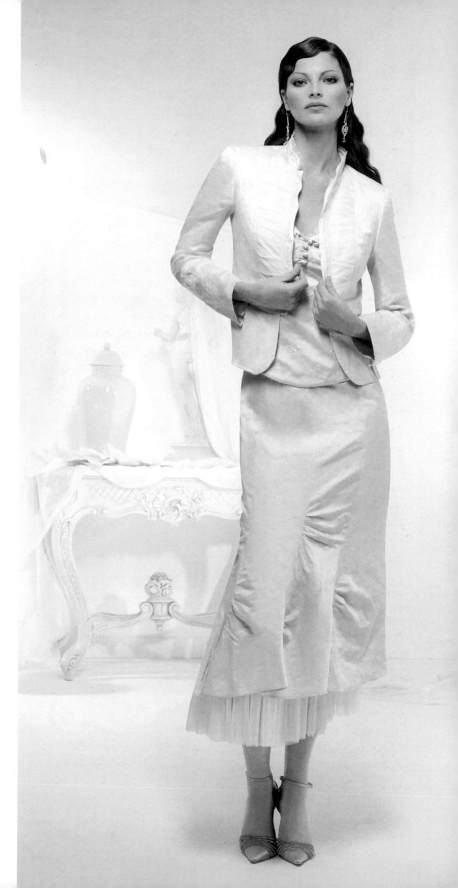

dresses

Neat hourglass With your balanced body line, the choice is yours. You may need to take your proportions into consideration to achieve a balanced look.

Full hourglass Choose a dress style that is soft and fluid. The ideal is the wrap or bias-cut dress that will drape.

Triangle A dress is not a good option for you, as finding the right fit will be difficult. Consider separates instead.

Inverted triangle A shift dress in a crisp fabric will be a good choice for you. The lines of the dress need some structure, and hip details (such as pockets) will work well.

Column Choose a dress that has slight waist emphasis, such as a half-belt at the back.

Rectangle Make the most of your straight lines by wearing a simple shift dress in luxury fabric. Details should be kept simple to keep your silhouette straight and uncluttered.

BELOW *The 1920s flapper dress is great for a woman without too many curves.*

VINTAGE DRESSES

You may be lucky enough to have the opportunity of wearing a family dress, or be able to buy a vintage outfit that will be unique to you. If you are keen to recycle a dress already worn or to acquire one from an antique or second-hand store, you may need to have it altered to fit — half a century or so ago, women were generally much smaller. Alternatively, you can incorporate pieces of the vintage dress into a new one: lace and other embellishments can be transferred by a dressmaker or tailor.

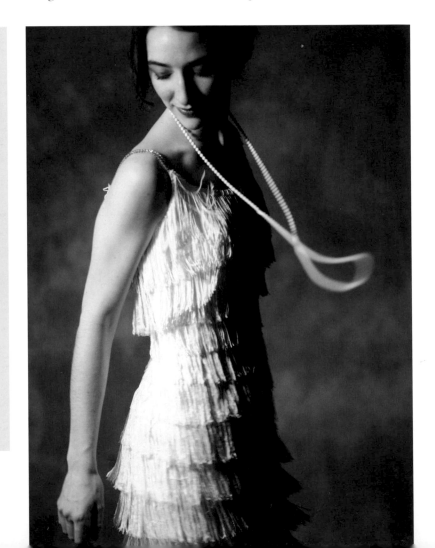

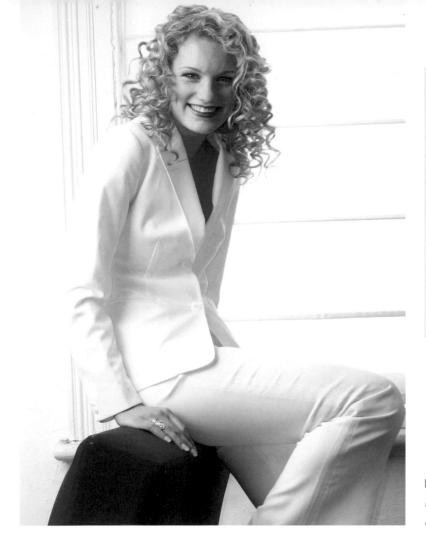

REMEMBER...

With all outfits – skirts, trousers, jackets, coats or dresses – check that the hemline does not fall at the widest point on your body. If you choose a patterned fabric, make sure it balances with your scale: a small bone structure needs small patterns; a large bone structure can take more dramatic designs.

LEFT *A white trouser suit in a luxury fabric is a good option for an informal wedding.*

trousers

Neat hourglass A fitted, flat-fronted trouser style with a waistband is best for you. If you have long legs, consider a turn-up/cuffs for added detail.

Full hourglass Select trousers without a front crease down the leg and avoid a front zip. Soft, fluid fabrics work well for you. Avoid details such as pockets and embellishments over the hip area.

Triangle A bootleg-style trouser will help to balance your hips. Avoid any pockets and other details, and keep your trousers simple.

Inverted triangle Straight or bootleg trousers with a crease down the front of the leg are ideal for you. You can choose to have pockets and embellishments on the hip area.

Column You need trousers with a crease down the front of the leg. Textured fabrics are good and you can do pockets successfully. Avoid wide-leg palazzo style.

Rectangle Your trousers should come without a waistband and be flat fronted with a side zip. You'll need a crease down the front of the leg if the trousers are formal. Softer styles work well for a more feminine look. If you opt for an elasticated band, make sure it doesn't show.

making the final choice

BEFORE ENTERING THE WORLD OF WEDDING DRESS STORES, A LITTLE FORETHOUGHT AND PLANNING WILL ENSURE YOU ENJOY THE EXPERIENCE *AND* GET EXACTLY WHAT YOU WANT AND WHAT SUITS YOU BEST. WITH THE KNOWLEDGE YOU HAVE ACQUIRED SO FAR FROM THIS BOOK, THERE IS NO NEED TO BE INTIMIDATED BY SALES PEOPLE. BE PREPARED TO TRY ON A RANGE OF DIFFERENT DRESSES, BECAUSE UNTIL YOU DO YOU REALLY WON'T KNOW WHAT WORKS AND WHAT DOESN'T.

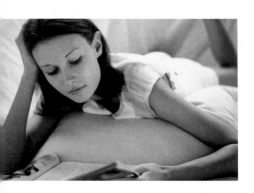

ABOVE *Make time to go through magazines to check out what the trends are and what is available at various price brackets.*

planning and research

As soon as you begin looking through wedding (and perhaps celebrity) magazines, you will find yourself overwhelmed by the choice available. Begin by tearing out pages that depict the styles of wedding dress to which you aspire.

Another source of inspiration is the internet, where you can research styles from around the world as well as discover what may be on your doorstep. You can also make a list of what you liked and disliked at weddings you have attended. All this may help to narrow your choice of options, although an exact replica of your friend's or a celebrity's wedding dress is probably not a good idea and demonstrates a lack of creativity.

Doing your research will give you some indication of a realistic budget, although you may find you have to spend a little more to get exactly what you want.

going shopping

If you can, take a day or two off from work during the week, as Saturday is a busy day and you may not get the attention that you want. Some stores prefer you to make an appointment. Don't go shopping when you are pre-menstrual and feeling bloated – choose a time when you are feeling good and confident about yourself.

Selecting a wedding dress or outfit is not a rush job. Take your time, visit as many stores as you can, and don't be too hasty in reaching your decision. Take

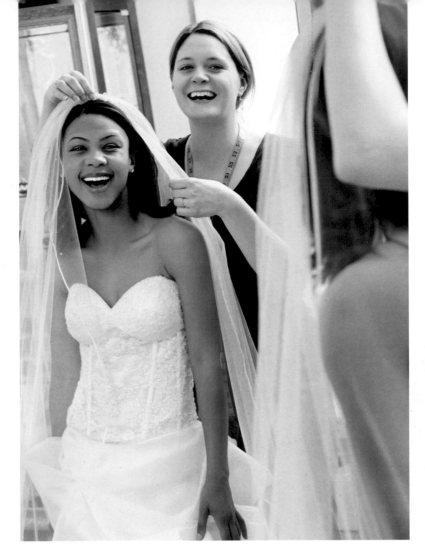

along someone you can trust – mother, friend or even a personal shopper who you know will give you unbiased and honest advice. Be prepared for your mother to shed a tear or two each time you step out of the changing room!

trying it on

On the day of your shopping trip, make sure you are happy with your appearance, with your hair done and a little make-up applied. Wear good underwear that you know gives you the support and shape you want. Take a selection of shoes with different heel heights so you can check their effect on the dress.

If you are not accustomed to wearing a long skirt, you will need to think about how you are going to walk and sit (and perhaps even kneel), and try all these activities while wearing the dresses. At the wedding, you will be seen alongside the groom, so take his stature into consideration when selecting the volume of your dress.

Think about practicalities. Will you be dressing on your own? Is the dress suitable for getting in and out of the car in which you will be travelling? How easy will it be to answer the call of nature? If you will be dancing the night away, can that beautiful long train be bustled up quickly and easily?

Finally, remember to try on veils and headdresses (see pages 84–85) at the same time to ensure they all work together.

ABOVE *Taking a close friend with you when choosing your dress can be great fun and is part of the ritual of being a bride-to-be.*

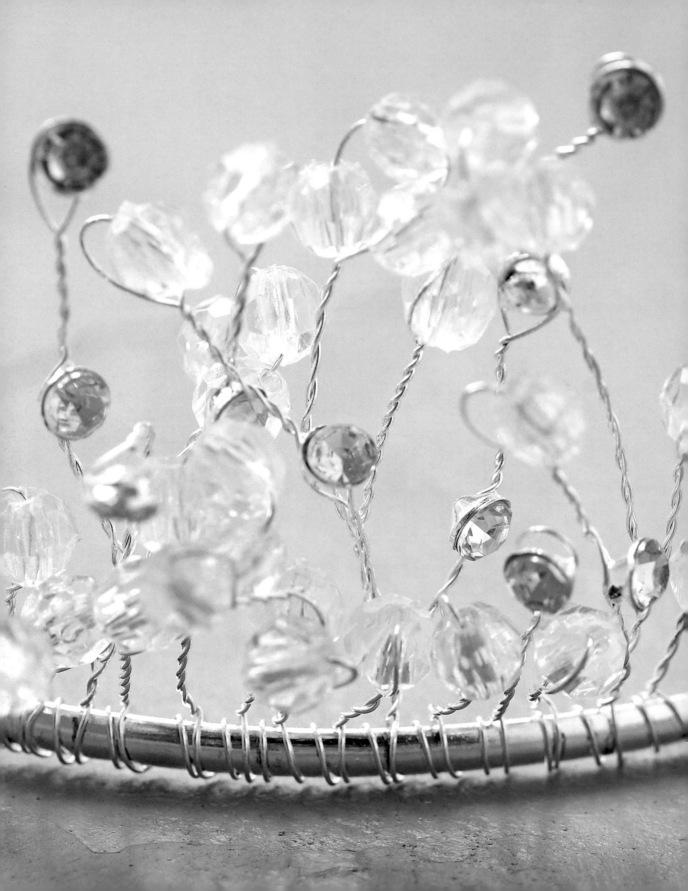

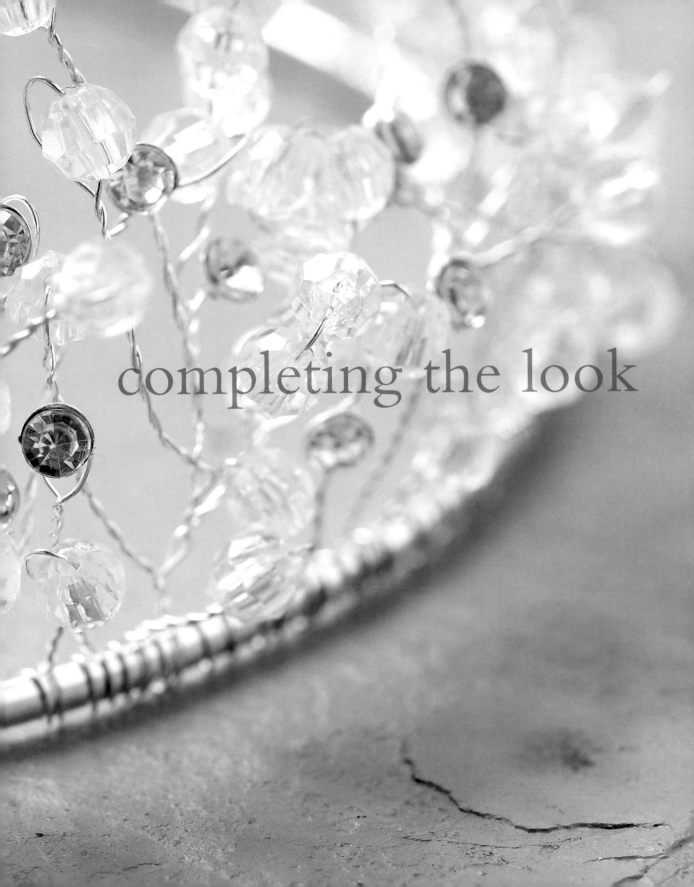

completing the look

your face shape

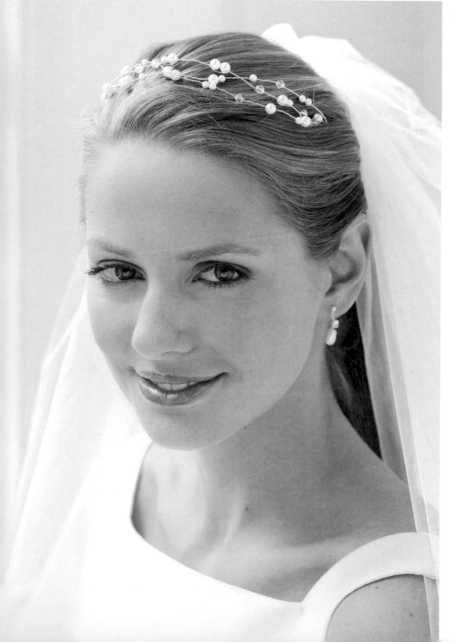

a perfect picture

To look beautiful from all aspects, you will need to make sure that your hair, veil, headdress and jewellery all work well with your face shape. You need to plan for the way your hair is styled, where you place your headdress, and how the veil is attached and falls, in order for all these elements to work together to achieve a well-balanced look and the perfect head shot. Remember to take your headdress and veil with you to the hairdresser when you go for a practice run.

LEFT *An oval face shape can wear any style of headdress and veil.*

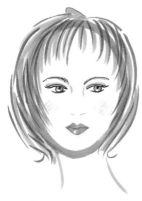

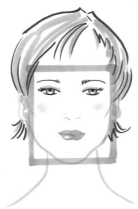

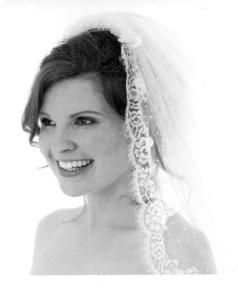

oval

You have balanced features and slightly rounded cheeks that narrow down to the jaw line. Your chin may be slightly pointed or rounded and your forehead is narrower than your cheekbones.

square

Your whole face looks angled. The width and length are basically equal. Your jaw line is straight and in line with your cheekbones, and your forehead is quite square.

ABOVE *A square-shaped face is flattered by having a fuller hairstyle at the temples.*

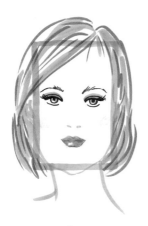

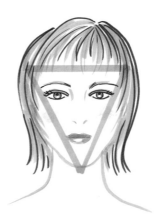

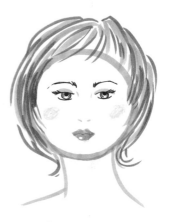

rectangle

Your face appears narrow, with the length greater than the width. Your forehead is high but square and your jaw line is angled. Your cheekbones may be pronounced.

inverted triangle

You have a wide forehead and your jaw line is much narrower than your cheekbones. Your chin appears a little pointed.

round

Your face is narrower at the forehead, fuller at the cheekbones and rounded down to the jaw line. Your cheeks are full and your whole face has a soft appearance.

oval

YOUR OVAL FACE SHAPE IS PERFECTLY BALANCED. THE ONLY CONSIDERATION TO TAKE INTO ACCOUNT IS WHETHER

YOU HAVE ANY FACIAL FEATURES THAT ARE NOT IN PROPORTION (SEE PAGES 86–87). HEADDRESSES AND

JEWELLERY ARE DESCRIBED IN DETAIL ON PAGES 83–85, MAKE-UP ON PAGES 119–124.

LONG HAIR UP
Look at the back of your head to see if it is nicely curved, in which case any style will do. If it is flat, a hairstyle with volume at the back will balance the shape.

LONG HAIR DOWN
Have your hair as natural or styled as you wish.

SHORT HAIR
To show off your face, avoid having too much hair coming forward on to your forehead.

HEADDRESS
A soft-line headdress is better for you than an angled style.

JEWELLERY
Your guidelines for size will depend on whether you are petite, average or grand in scale. Balance the dimensions of your jewellery to match.

MAKE-UP
Gently slant your eyebrows upwards at the end. Apply a hint of blusher around your temples and on the tip of your chin.

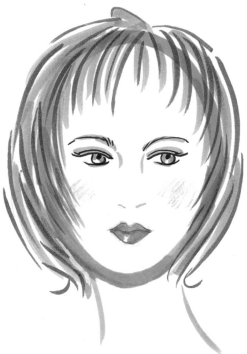

square

YOUR SQUARE-SHAPED FACE WILL BE ENHANCED BY ADDING SOFT CONTOURS WITH YOUR HAIRSTYLE AND
MAKE-UP APPLICATION. WHICHEVER WAY YOU DECIDE TO WEAR YOUR HAIR, TRY TO ACHIEVE SOME FULLNESS
AT THE SIDES TO GIVE THE ILLUSION OF A MORE OVAL-SHAPED FACE.

LONG HAIR UP

If you are putting your hair up,
you will need to add width to
the sides of your temples. Either
back-comb your hair here
before pulling it back, or keep
some hair loose around the
temples to achieve this balance.

LONG HAIR DOWN

Try a layered cut with
feathering on to your face,
which will soften its outline.

SHORT HAIR

A rounded, layered cut with
volume on the sides of the
temples will be perfect for
you. Avoid a one-length bob
finishing at the jaw line,
with a straight fringe.

HEADDRESS

Crown, tiara or wreath styles
will soften the sharp angles of
your face.

JEWELLERY

Avoid geometric styles: instead,
select softer, rounder shapes.

MAKE-UP

Apply darker shading on your
jaw line and keep the line of
your blusher curved.

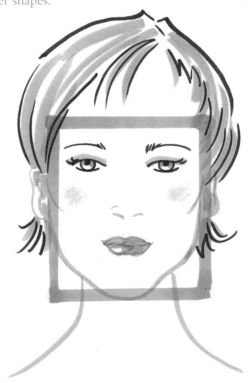

rectangle

WITH THIS SHAPE, THE OVERALL IDEA IS TO CREATE THE ILLUSION THAT YOU HAVE A SHORTER FACE. THIS MAY BE ACHIEVED IN MANY DIFFERENT WAYS BUT SOME SORT OF FRINGE OVER THE FOREHEAD WILL ALWAYS HELP. IF YOU HAVE A LONG NECK CONSIDER A CHOKER-STYLE NECKLACE OR A DRESS WITH SOME FORM OF COLLAR.

LONG HAIR UP

A fringe will be perfect for you. Wear the bulk of your hair at the nape of your neck rather than on the top, which would further elongate your face.

LONG HAIR DOWN

Keep your fringe and have your hair layered to soften your face. Avoid a centre parting.

SHORT HAIR

Choose a layered style, flicked out to add width to your face.

HEADDRESS

A Juliet cap will keep the length of your face to a minimum; alternatively, a narrow tiara would also be good. A fascinator slanted on the side will add width to your face.

JEWELLERY

Your earrings will need to add width to your face, so avoid long, dangling styles. Also avoid long chain necklaces.

MAKE-UP

Bring your eye shadow outwards and upwards to give width to your face. Define your blusher closer to the hair and outer cheekbones.

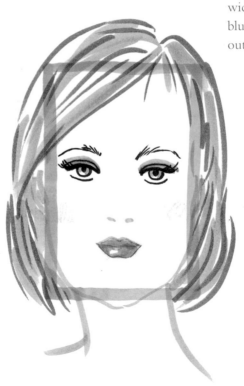

inverted triangle

BY ADDING VOLUME AND INTEREST TO YOUR JAW LINE YOU CAN GIVE THE ILLUSION OF A NARROWER FOREHEAD AND CHEEKBONES. THINK CAREFULLY ABOUT THE CHOICE OF NECKLINE ON YOUR WEDDING DRESS. A DEEP V WILL ONLY EMPHASIZE YOUR NARROW CHIN. A SCOOP OR ROUNDED NECKLINE WILL BE MORE FLATTERING.

LONG HAIR UP

You need soft curls to fall from all around the hairline of a swept-up style.

LONG HAIR DOWN

A flicked-out, layered style will add width around your jaw line.

SHORT HAIR

A feathered, rounded fringe will soften your forehead. You'll need volume at the jaw line – your hair can be flicked under or out.

HEADDRESS

Choose a headdress style that can be worn at the back of your head, or try individual pins or small combs.

JEWELLERY

Dangling earrings with interest at the bottom are perfect for you. If you choose to wear studs, balance them with an interesting necklace if your dress can take it.

MAKE-UP

Make your lips the focal point of your face, using a lipgloss over your lipstick. Apply blusher to the apple of your cheeks.

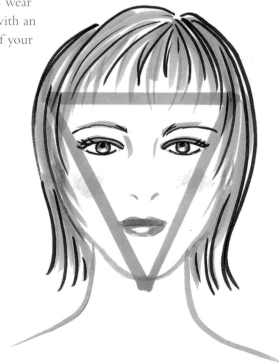

round

YOUR ROUND, FEMININE FACE IS THE PERFECT CANVAS FOR SLIGHTLY MORE ANGLED HAIRSTYLES AND MAKE-UP

APPLICATIONS. ALTHOUGH YOU MAY WANT TO HAVE YOUR LONG HAIR PULLED UP, THIS WILL ONLY MAKE YOUR

FACE LOOK ROUNDER, SO TRY A STYLE WHERE SOME OF YOUR HAIR FALLS ON TO YOUR FACE.

LONG HAIR UP
A French pleat will give a slightly elongated look to your head, ensuring you have some volume at the top.

LONG HAIR DOWN
An asymmetrical parting and fringe work particularly well if you are wearing your hair down and loose.

SHORT HAIR
A feathered style coming forward on to your face will suit you best.

HEADDRESS
A slightly taller or angled tiara or headdress will be perfect.

JEWELLERY
Neat-fitting earrings are best for you – avoid hoops.

MAKE-UP
Keep your eyebrows as straight as possible. Use a highlighter straight along your cheekbones to create some contour.

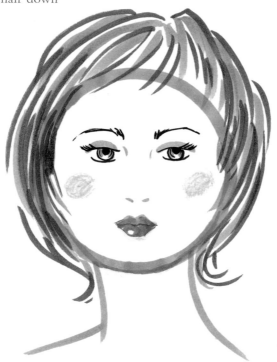

jewellery

FOR YOUR WEDDING, JEWELLERY SHOULD BE KEPT TO A MINIMUM SO THAT IT IS YOU WHO SHINES ON THE DAY. YOUR CHOICE OF JEWELLERY WILL DEPEND ON THE STYLE OF YOUR DRESS AND YOUR PROPORTIONS. YOU MAY EVEN DECIDE TO WEAR A FABULOUS FAMILY HEIRLOOM.

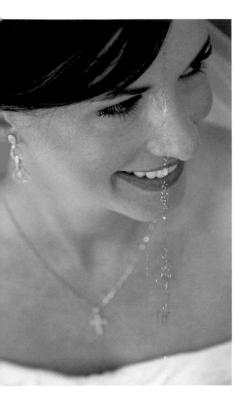

ABOVE *Keep your jewellery simple to avoid detracting from your wedding dress.*

RIGHT *You may choose to wear a matching comb in your hair.*

earrings

• Small or stud-style earrings will suit all. These can be diamonds, pearls or any other gemstones.

• Drop or dangling earrings are best worn with your hair away from your face – really long ones require a long neck.

necklaces

Necklaces should be chosen with the neckline of your dress in mind: the lower the neckline, the more detailed your necklace can be.

• If your bodice is heavily embellished, a simple necklace is best, or none at all.

• A choker requires a long neck and low neckline.

bracelets and watches

• If your dress has long sleeves, do not clutter your wrists with bracelets and a watch.

• If you want to wear a watch, choose one that is jewelled.

rings

• Wear only your engagement ring, but not on your ring finger. Transfer it to the third finger of your right hand, so that your ring finger is free to receive your wedding ring. You can slip your engagement ring back on after the ceremony.

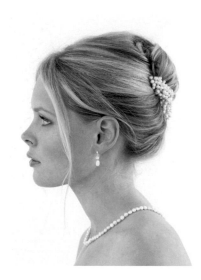

headdresses and veils

A HEADDRESS AND VEIL WILL COMPLETE YOUR OVERALL LOOK. CHOOSING THE RIGHT ONES FOR YOU DEPENDS ON YOUR PERSONAL STYLE AND PREFERENCES, AS WELL AS THE DRESS YOU WILL BE WEARING. YOU'LL ALSO NEED TO THINK ABOUT THE HAIRSTYLE YOU WANT ON THE DAY, TO ENSURE THAT EVERYTHING WORKS IN HARMONY.

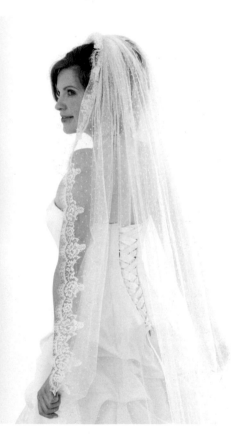

ABOVE *This cathedral spotted net veil is trimmed with scalloped edge lace for a romantic look.*

headdresses

Tiara Jewelled or beaded semi-circle of various heights, worn on top of the head towards the front. A tiara will give height to your face or forehead and can be rounded or angled, depending on the shape of your face. A rounded shape will soften an angled face (square or rectangle), while an angular tiara will give contours to a round face.

Crown Jewelled or beaded full circle of various heights, worn on top of the head. A crown will add height to any face, so avoid it if you have a rectangle face shape.

Alice band Band of various widths that fits closely to the head and is tucked behind the ears. It can be jewelled, beaded or covered in the same fabric as used for your dress. An Alice band is good for all face shapes except inverted triangle.

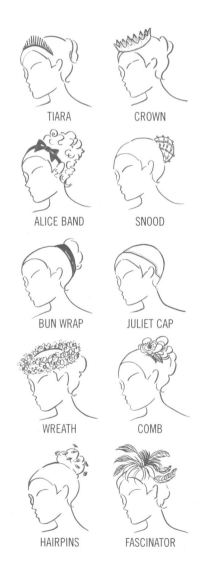

TIARA

CROWN

ALICE BAND

SNOOD

BUN WRAP

JULIET CAP

WREATH

COMB

HAIRPINS

FASCINATOR

Snood Decorated net that encases your hair at the back of your head. Avoid a snood if you have a short neck as it sits low on the back of the head.

Bun wrap Decoration with which to wrap you hair if you are wearing it up in a bun. The wrap can be decorated with beads or sequins to co-ordinate with your dress. Worn on the back of the head, it is particularly good if the back of your head is flat.

Juliet cap Small, circular, decorated cap that fits on top of your head, to which a train can be attached. It works best with a long neck.

Wreath Crown-like garland made from fresh or silk flowers that rests on the head. A wreath is particularly good if you have a high forehead or rectangular face. It is best avoided if you have a low forehead or an especially round face.

Comb Available in various sizes and depths either to decorate or to keep your hair and veil in place. A comb will keep a section of hair secure as the long teeth grip well. It can be embellished with flowers or beads.

Hairpins Single pieces of decoration to be scattered throughout the hairstyle for a relaxed look.

Fascinator Small cap decorated with all sizes of feathers, ribbons and flowers, worn slightly on the side of the head. Make sure you have enough hair for the fascinator to sit firmly and securely in it – elastic bands at the back of your hair is not a good look!

veils

The volume and the length of your veil will depend on your height and the line of your dress. Also take into account how formal your wedding is. Traditionally some ceremonies call for the bride to wear a veil which is often removed for the celebrations afterwards.

Fly away Informal veil that reaches to the shoulders and can be multi-layered.

Elbow Veil that reaches to the elbow.

Finger tip Veil that falls to the tip of the fingers.

Double tier Two-layered veil in which the shorter layer is worn over the face during the first part of the ceremony, if desired. The second layer, which can be of any length, remains at the back.

Chapel Veil that reaches the bottom of the dress.

Cathedral Longest and most dramatic of all veils, falling on to the floor behind the dress.

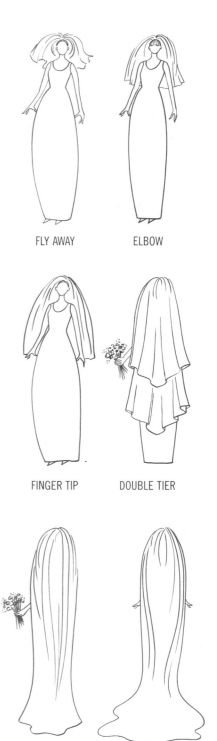

FLY AWAY   ELBOW

FINGER TIP   DOUBLE TIER

CHAPEL   CATHEDRAL

disguise and hide:
questions and answers

SOMETIMES THERE MAY BE ASPECTS OF YOUR FACE OR BODY YOU ARE UNHAPPY ABOUT. BY CLEVER USE OF

MAKE-UP, HAIRSTYLE AND ACCESSORIES THESE CAN BE MINIMIZED, TO CREATE THE EFFECT YOU WANT.

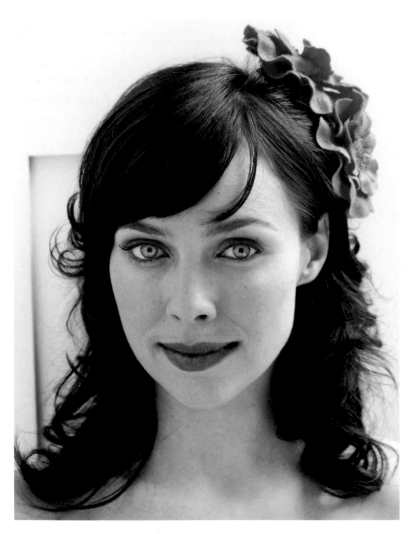

Q *I have protruding ears. How can I ensure they don't show?*

A You will need to use your hair to help hide your ears. If you choose to wear your hair up, you will need loose sections of hair falling in front of them. Long hair needs volume at the sides so that your ears are covered, and short hair should be styled with the same aim. Choose a headdress and veil that are positioned on top of your head rather than on the sides.

Q *I have a very high forehead: what are my options for my hair and headdress?*

A If possible, choose a hairstyle with a fringe as this will

LEFT *A full or partial fringe with a side parting will help to disguise a full forehead or a rectangular face.*

immediately disguise your high forehead. You do not want a headdress that adds height, so a wreath (sitting on top of the forehead if you do not have a fringe), narrow tiara or Alice band will be perfect. Keep your veil close to the top of your head, with volume at the back or sides.

Q *I have very fine hair and need to know how to wear it at my wedding, as well as how to attach a veil and headdress to it.*

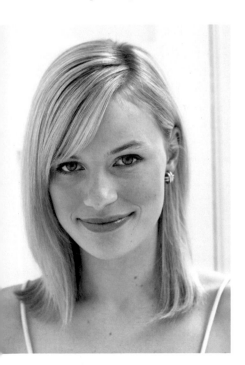

A If you have long hair, wearing it in a bun will provide volume and give you somewhere to position your headdress, which can then be used to attach the veil. However, wearing you hair short will give you more headdress options. These need to grip your head rather than your hair, so selecting a tiara, wreath or Alice band will give you the base to which to attach your veil.

Q *What can I do to disguise my rather large nose?*

A Apply a darker shade of foundation all over your nose, then use a highlighter along your cheekbones and on the tip of your chin to bring out these areas. Details and volume at the back of your head will counterbalance your nose. Avoid a centre parting at all costs.

Q *What do I do to disguise my double chin?*

A Choose an open neckline on the bodice of your dress. Powder the whole of your neck area with a dark shade of powder or bronzer, and draw attention away from the area by bringing interest and focus to your eyes. Avoid shoulder-length hairstyles and veils.

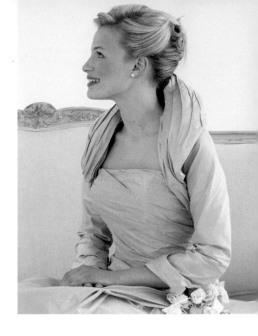

Q *I have very prominent collarbones: what do I do?*

A For a cold-weather wedding, choose a dress with a high collar if you have a long neck. If you have a short neck, make sure you select a neckline that hides your collarbones (see pages 62–63). For a warm-weather wedding, an insert of lace, organza or other lightweight sheer fabric will camouflage your collarbones. Embellishments, such as beading or embroidery, on the bodice of your dress will distract attention from your upper chest and collarbones.

wraps, jackets and coats

YOU MAY FEEL YOU NEED TO COVER UP FOR PART OR ALL OF THE WEDDING. THE VENUE MAY DEMAND THIS, AND IF YOU ARE HAVING A WINTER WEDDING YOU WILL WANT TO KEEP WARM. THE CHOICE IS DOWN TO YOUR PERSONAL PREFERENCE, THE STYLE OF YOUR WEDDING DRESS AND YOUR BUDGET. FABRICS WILL RANGE FROM FAKE FUR OR VELVET TO LACE AND THE LIGHTEST SHEER FABRICS.

shrug

A shrug is ideal for wearing during the ceremony if you have chosen a strapless dress or if your upper arms and shoulders are not your best feature.

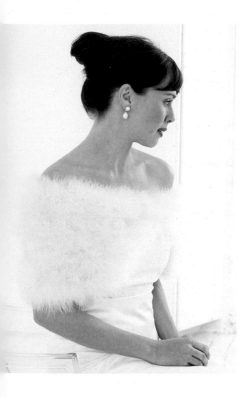

bolero

A bolero gives the same coverage as the shrug but is more structured and often a garment in its own right.

jacket

A jacket is the ideal solution for a cool-weather wedding and allows for the dress shape to be seen and admired.

coat

A wedding dress with a matching coat is a very elegant solution for winter weddings. Often the coat is embellished and the dress underneath is simpler in style.

stole

A stole can be made from many different types of fabric, from sheer lace to feathers and fake fur. Make sure that it stays in place as you move around.

cape

A cape can be short or full length. You could use it as an alternative way of adding colour to a winter wedding.

LEFT *A fun furry stole will add glamour to your wedding dress.*

BELOW *A ribbon lace jacket gives ample coverage, while maintaing a sheer look.*

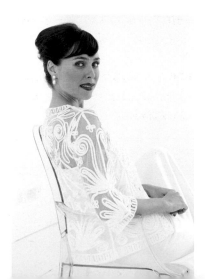

shoes

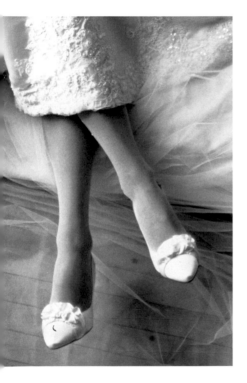

style and colour

The style of footwear you choose depends on the dress you wear, the venue and your personality. If you want to take the opportunity to try something unusual, it is often easiest to do so by choosing 'different' footwear, be it a pair of colourful ballet shoes or pink cowboy boots.

Don't forget to try your dress with your shoes to ensure the length is correct, and practise walking in them while wearing the dress. If you have chosen a coloured gown, you can have the shoes dyed to match the dress.

put comfort first

You may want to select a type of shoe in which you already know how to walk comfortably. If you have never worn a particular style, choose a different one unless you are prepared to practise. Although you may want to wear a stunning pair of stilettos, make sure you have a second pair of more sensible shoes to hand in case your feet give up. Whatever footwear you choose, break it in before the big day. Wear your shoes around the house, scuff the soles and make sure there are no hard edges on them that will blister your feet.

ABOVE *Remember to test-drive your shoes before the big day.*

RIGHT *To add drama, why not wear a colourful pair of heels? In your colours of course.*

FAR RIGHT *Add a little glitz for glamour as you walk down the aisle.*

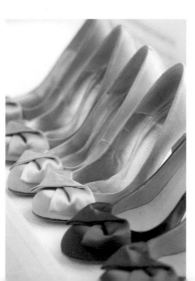

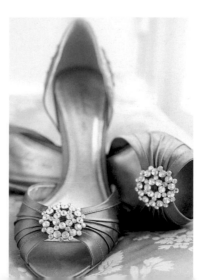

the bridal bouquet

YOUR BOUQUET WILL COMPLETE YOUR LOOK AS YOU WALK DOWN THE AISLE, BRINGING TOGETHER YOUR PERSONALITY AND THE COLOUR THEME OF YOUR WEDDING. YOU MUST ALSO ENSURE THAT THE BOUQUET STYLE COMPLEMENTS YOUR DRESS, BODY SHAPE AND SCALE.

making your choice

The range of bouquets available can be overwhelming, but by following the advice given here and overleaf you will be able to select an appropriate and manageable bouquet. Your flowers do not necessarily have to be fresh: silk flowers will provide a lasting memory of your wedding day.

colour

The choice of colour for your bouquet needs to harmonize with that of your wedding dress. This can be either tonal or contrasting. See pages 12–17 for the best accent colours for your dominant palette.

basic shapes

Bear in mind your scale when choosing the size of your bouquet to make sure that the overall look is in proportion.

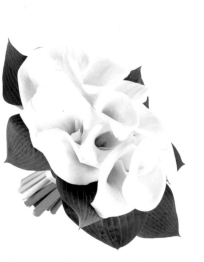

Posy Small, round bouquet that is good for petite brides.

Nosegay Medium-sized, round bouquet that is tied tightly for ease of carrying.

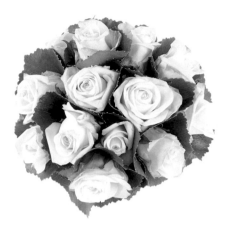

Round Full bouquet with larger blooms than a nosegay. It is often mixed with some smaller flowers.

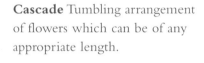

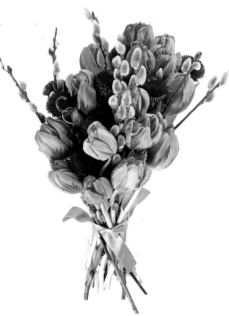

Cascade Tumbling arrangement of flowers which can be of any appropriate length.

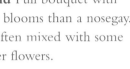

Hand tied More informal bouquet, often tied with a ribbon. Also known as a spray.

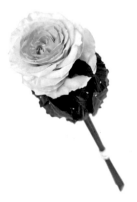

Pageant Bouquet of long-stemmed flowers, often carried over the arm.

Single Single 'statement' flower. The stem can be ribboned or decorated. Can be decorated with ribbons, bows or jewels.

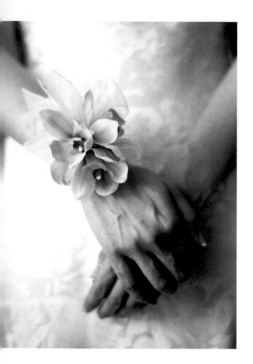

ABOVE *A floral wristband is a simple yet elegant alternative to a traditional bouquet.*

style and scale

Your bouquet should tie in with any theme you might have for the day. A relaxed and informal wedding will call for a hand-tied bouquet or even a single flower, while a formal occasion will demand a constructed bouquet such as a nosegay.

The types of flowers you use will also be part of your theme. For example, less formal flowers, such as a hand-tied bouquet with cottage-garden style flowers, will work well for a summer wedding, or choose berries and grasses for an autumn (fall) ceremony.

Whatever the style or time of year for your wedding, you must also consider your own scale. If you have a petite build, a smaller bouquet with dainty flowers will suit you perfectly; larger, more dramatic blooms will create a balanced look for a grander scale bride.

complementing your dress

Shift This simple style of dress, best for straight body lines, will benefit from a simple-shaped bouquet such as a hand tied using only a couple of different flowers in similar tones.

Empire With this dress, most of the attention will be on the top half. This gives you the opportunity to hold your bouquet below the bust line, so a cascade will bring detail to the body of the dress.

Bias cut The flowing lines of a bias-cut dress are beautifully enhanced with a pageant-style bouquet or simple single stem statement flower.

Fishtail With details on the hemline of this dress, a posy or round-style bouquet will draw attention to the waistline.

A-line The A-line dress is so versatile that all styles of bouquet will work well.

Ball gown To make the most of your wonderful full skirt, ensure the bouquet is the focus of your waist with a nosegay or larger round arrangement.

completing the picture

If you are having bridesmaids you may want them to have the same shape bouquet as you, but with different flowers in toning colours. Equally you could go for something completely different. Your groom's buttonhole should complement one or two of the flowers in your bouquet.

RIGHT *This soft bride's dress is enhanced by carrying some creamy white peonies to co-ordinate with the white embroidery.*

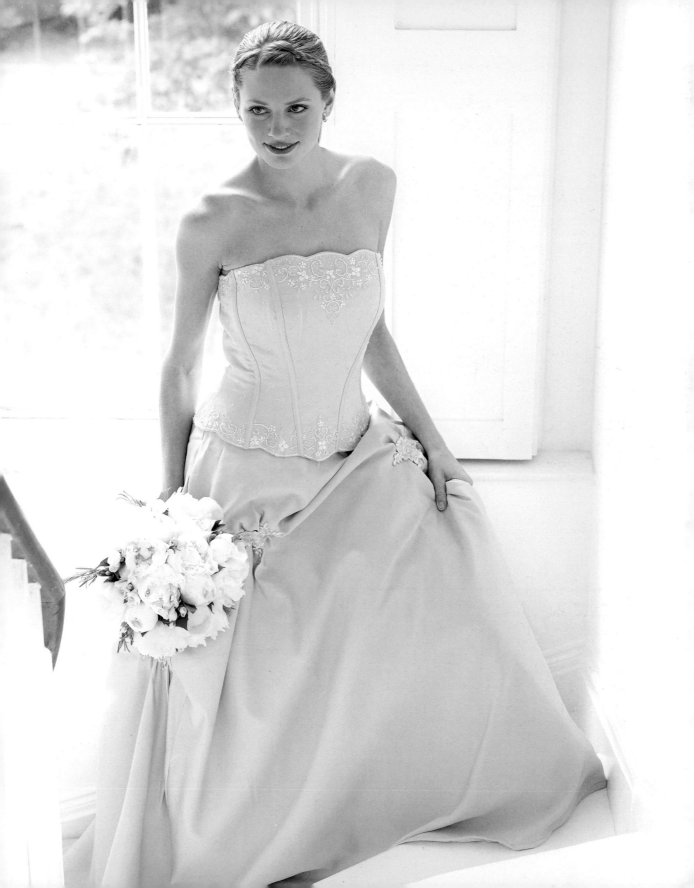

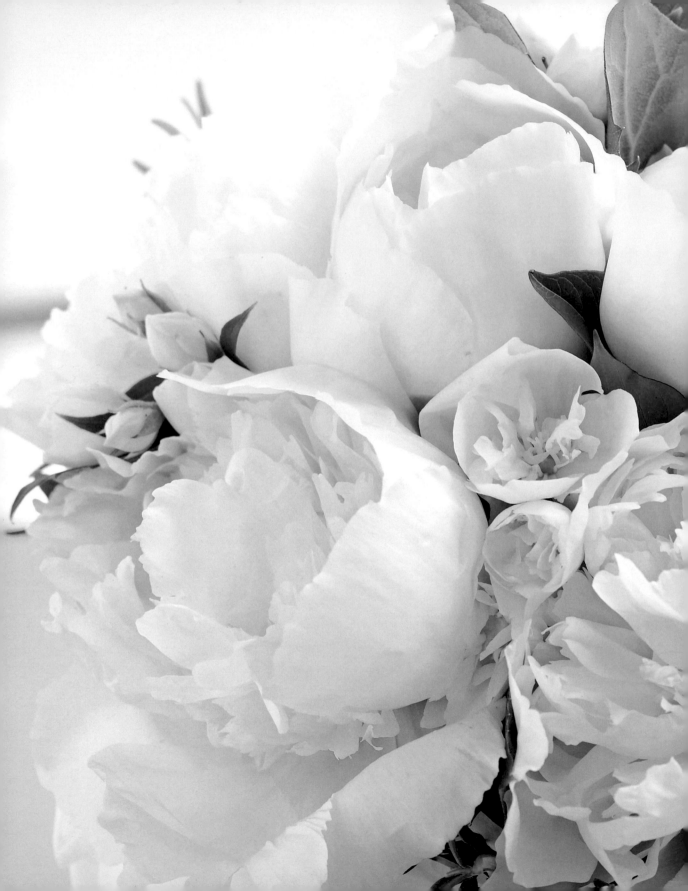

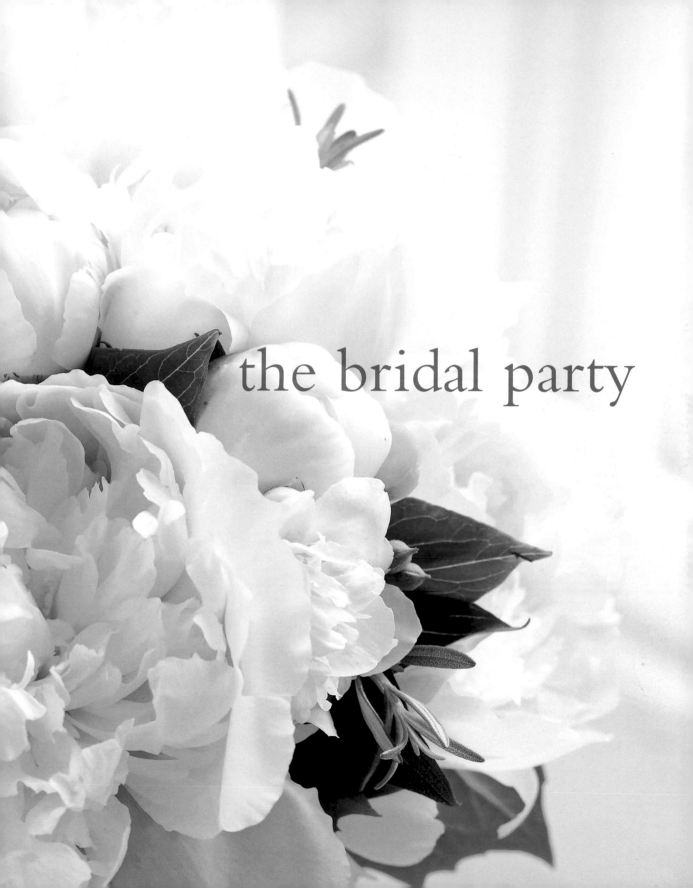

the bridal party

bridesmaids' dresses: colours

IT IS AN HONOUR TO BE A BRIDESMAID, AND OFTEN THOSE YOU HAVE ASKED WILL BE AS EXCITED AS YOU ARE.

SHOPPING FOR BRIDESMAIDS' OUTFITS CAN BE A FUN EXPERIENCE FOR YOU ALL, ALTHOUGH YOU WILL NEED

A CLEAR IDEA OF WHAT YOU WANT THEM TO LOOK LIKE BECAUSE THEY WILL FRAME YOU IN YOUR WEDDING

PHOTOGRAPHS. HAPPY BRIDESMAIDS MAKE GOOD PHOTOGRAPHS, SO ENSURING THEY ARE COMFORTABLE IN

WHAT THEY ARE WEARING WILL GUARANTEE EVERYONE IS RADIANT ON THE DAY.

colours for all

If you are having only one bridesmaid, the choice of colour is easier because you simply need to choose one that suits her and complements your colour scheme (see pages 12–17). With more than one bridesmaid, the choice can be more challenging. One might be a redhead, another a blonde and another dark haired: what is going to suit them all?

It is actually possible to choose a colour that works well for all your bridesmaids. In the **colour me beautiful** colour system there are shades that are universal and will suit everyone, whatever their colouring.

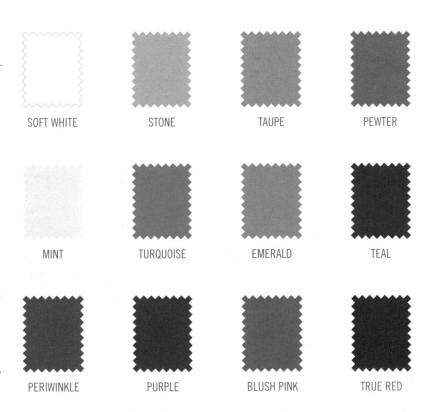

SOFT WHITE	STONE	TAUPE	PEWTER
MINT	TURQUOISE	EMERALD	TEAL
PERIWINKLE	PURPLE	BLUSH PINK	TRUE RED

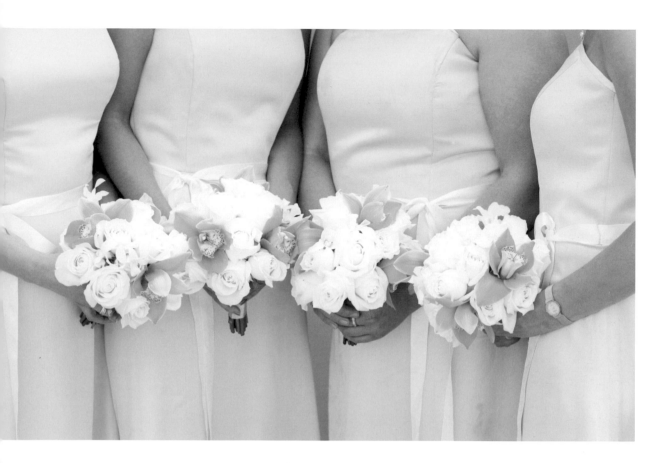

ABOVE *Against the light colour of the bridesmaids' dresses, the choice of light flowers blend and balance the overall look.*

LEFT *The striking purple of these bridesmaids' dresses is picked out in the bouquets of brightly coloured and contrasting flowers.*

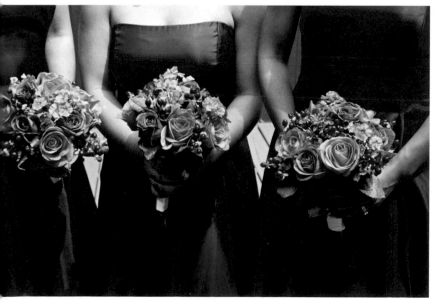

the right shade

The alternative to choosing a universal colour is to have a colour theme for your bridesmaids, whereby they each wear a shade of the colour that suits them best. In this way, you can achieve a stunning look for your bridal party.

The choice of colour theme will often be determined by the time of year. Pastels work well in spring or summer, reds and greens in winter. Purples, aquas and blues will look good all year round.

By following the suggestions opposite you will achieve a colourful and happy group. Selecting colours in this way will also work when you have a mix of adults and children.

BELOW *Bridesmaids do not have to wear the same style or colour of dress, as long as both the shape and the colour of their dresses suit them and complement each other.*

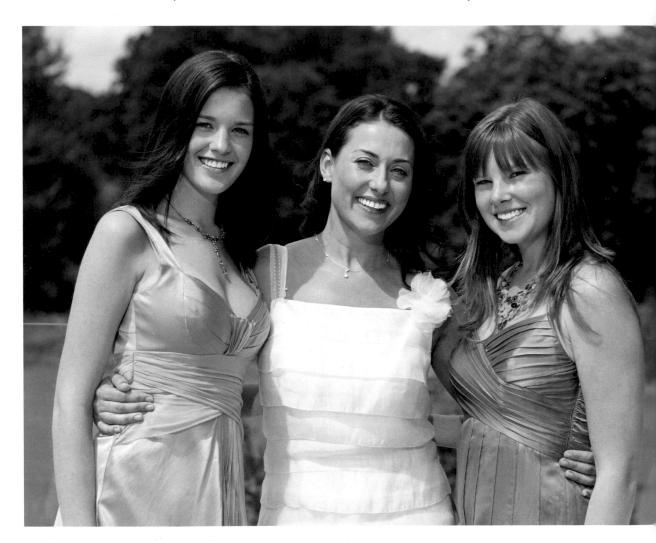

	LIGHT	DEEP	WARM	COOL	CLEAR	SOFT
PASTELS	LIGHT APRICOT	PRIMROSE	APRICOT	ICY VIOLET	SKY BLUE	MINT
BLUES	SKY BLUE	TRUE BLUE	LIGHT PERIWINKLE	CORNFLOWER	CHINESE BLUE	SAPPHIRE
GREENS	APPLE GREEN	FOREST	MOSS	BLUE-GREEN	EVERGREEN	VERBENA
AQUAS	LIGHT AQUA	TEAL	TURQUOISE	PEPPERMINT	LIGHT TEAL	JADE
PURPLES	VIOLET	ROYAL PURPLE	PURPLE	LIGHT PERIWINKLE	BRIGHT PERIWINKLE	SOFT VIOLET
PINKS	PASTEL PINK	BURGUNDY	CORAL	ROSE PINK	HOT PINK	BLUSH PINK
REDS	GERANIUM	TRUE RED	ORANGE-RED	BLUE-RED	SCARLET	CLARET
BLACKS AND GREYS	LIGHT GREY	BLACK	GREY-GREEN	MEDIUM GREY	CHARCOAL	PEWTER

bridesmaids' dresses: shapes

WHEN YOU START TO THINK ABOUT DRESSES FOR YOUR BRIDESMAIDS, VISIT DEPARTMENT STORES AND HIGH STREET SHOPS AND CHECK THE INTERNET TO GATHER IDEAS AND INSPIRATION. KEEP THEIR SIZES, PERSONALITIES AND COLOURING IN MIND TO MAKE SURE YOU END UP WITH HAPPY AND RELAXED BRIDESMAIDS ON YOUR WEDDING DAY.

first considerations

You will need to consider the following points:

• If you pay for the bridesmaids' dresses, you will have a lot more say in the matter.

• If the bridesmaids are paying for themselves, let them have their say.

• You may want the dresses to have a life after the wedding, so you will all need to think about whether they can be worn again for other occasions. Choosing an evening dress from a high street store will make this a more feasible proposition.

• The fabric of the bridesmaids' dresses does not have to be as luxurious as yours. You could even choose the same style dress as yours but in a different fabric, such as cotton.

• You might want a patterned fabric, in which case it is important to bear in mind the scale of your bridesmaids and the size of the pattern.

one style suits all?

Each of your bridesmaids will, of course, have her own body shape. However, there are certain styles of dress that will work well for most:

A-line (especially if two-piece) Because this style of dress comes in many different formats it will be easier to accommodate all body shapes. The skirt can be fuller or narrower; the waistline on the waist or dropped.

Empire This dress will suit your bridesmaids whatever their age but in particular if you have children. It is also comfortable to wear for a long day. This dress can hide a multitude of sins and will work for the unexpected announcement from one of your bridesmaids a few months before the wedding that she is pregnant.

range of styles

You can still achieve a co-ordinated group by choosing different styles of dress to suit your bridesmaids' respective body shapes (see pages 46–47), but keeping the colour the same or choosing a colour theme. When making decisions, think about the fact that:

• The bridesmaids' dresses must not be more elaborate than your wedding dress.

• You may want to choose an embellishment to tie-in with your dress.

• If you choose a print, ensure that the colour co-ordinates with your dress and theme.

RIGHT *These bridesmaids stand out in rose pink in the same style of dress as the bride.*

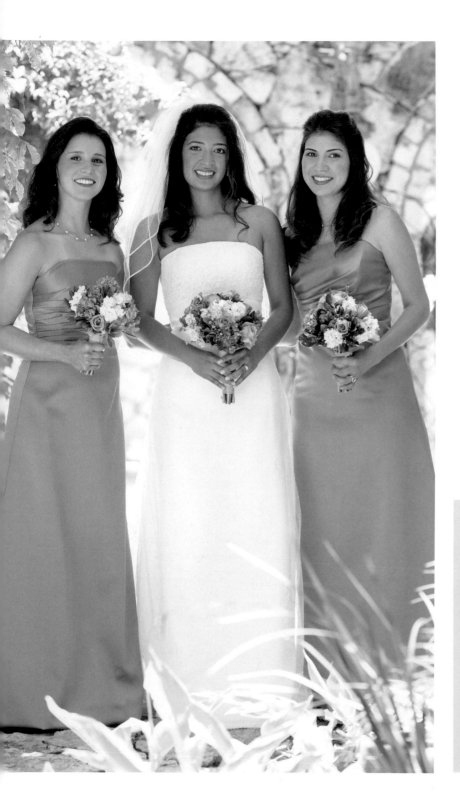

MAKING COMPROMISES

Don't dress your biker friend in a Barbie dress! This doesn't mean that she should come in jeans and Doc Marten boots, but a simple style of dress or separates will make her feel more at home. Everyone may have to compromise a little, but some forethought and planning will ensure no one is unhappy.

men's colours

DO NOT OVERLOOK THE MEN WHO WILL BE AT YOUR WEDDING. WHAT THEY CHOOSE (OR YOU TELL THEM) TO WEAR MUST COMPLEMENT WHAT YOU ARE WEARING AND BE CONSISTENT WITH THE REST OF THE BRIDAL PARTY. A LITTLE GUIDANCE ON COLOUR AND FIT WILL ENSURE THAT THEY, TOO, LOOK THE PART AND FEEL COMFORTABLE.

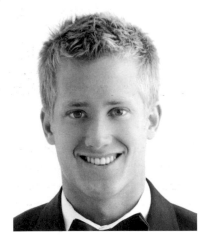

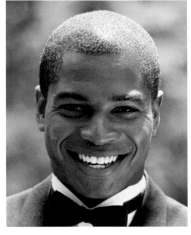

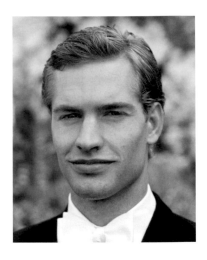

light

His look is pale and youthful, and he may even have a sensitive skin. His beard is light and his hair blond or minimal. He has blond eyebrows and lashes, and his eyes are pale blue, grey or pale green.

Don't overwhelm him with very dark colours: charcoal greys and light navy are best. If he has to wear dark colours, make sure his tie/cravat is in a light colour.

deep

His look is strong and definite. He has dark brown to black hair, and his facial hair is dark and prominent. His skin can be pale, through olive, to the darkest brown. He has deep, dark eyes.

Keep his colours strong and deep. A shirt in a contrasting colour is also good.

warm

He has an overall golden look consisting of ginger-blond, auburn or red hair. His skin is pale with freckles and his beard may grow gingery. His eyes are green, blue or brown, perhaps with yellow flecks in them.

Charcoal grey and navy are much better for him than black. Choose his shirt colour carefully: white will make him look as if he has been up all night, so go for soft white or cream.

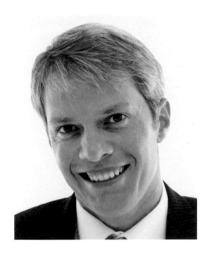

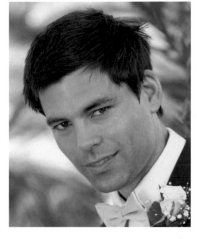

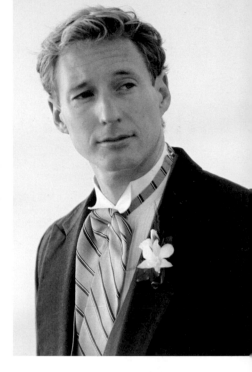

cool

His hair may be greying at the temples or completely grey, while his facial hair may be black with flecks of grey or white. He has rosy or pink tones to his skin if he is Caucasian, and a bluish-grey undertone if he is black. His eyes are blue, grey or cool brown.

Black works well, teamed with blues, pinks, lavenders and even burgundy. Avoid any browns or yellow-based colours.

clear

He has dark hair and bright, clear eyes that can be green, blue or brown. His complexion is often pale with dark eyebrows and lashes.

Because of his contrasting look he needs bright, clear colours to complement his striking appearance. Fabrics with a sheen work well as they reflect the light. Contrast his look between dark and light or bright colours.

muted

He has dark blond to medium-brown hair with eyebrows and lashes to match. His skin is light to olive with soft, blended tones in his eyes which can be blue, green or brown.

He needs to avoid high contrast and is much better in a blended, tonal look – woven, textured fabrics are perfect. Shantung ties and cravats work best. Avoid harsh contrasts: charcoal grey and soft white will be far more flattering than black and pure white.

men's body shapes

GETTING THE RIGHT SUIT OR OUTFIT FOR YOUR PARTNER IS NEARLY AS IMPORTANT AS CHOOSING YOUR OWN DRESS. IT'S NOT JUST A MATTER OF PURCHASING A SMART SUIT: MEN'S SUITS COME IN DIFFERENT SHAPES AND CUTS, SO IT IS IMPORTANT TO UNDERSTAND WHAT HIS BEST STYLE WILL BE. WHAT THE GROOM WEARS WILL DICTATE THE LOOK FOR THE REST OF THE MEN IN THE BRIDAL PARTY.

take a look

This is the fun bit. Get your man to strip off in front of you and have a good look at him. His body shape will dictate what are the best looks for him, be it the shape of his suit, the type of fabric or the pattern on his tie. You may also need to consider his proportions. For example, a man with short legs does not look good in wide trousers, while tapered trousers will give a long-legged man a beanpole appearance.

check the fit

• The collar of the jacket should fit against the collar of the shirt with no gap in between.
• Jacket sleeves should finish at the break of the wrist, allowing 1.5 cm (¾ in) of shirt to show below the jacket sleeve.
• For a good fit the waistband of the trouser should sit as near to the navel as possible.
• The trouser legs should fall with one break only across the shoe.

BELOW *Details such as real button holes on jackets, double cuffs and cufflinks all add to the glamour of the day.*

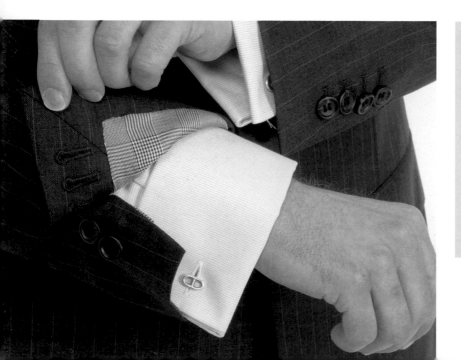

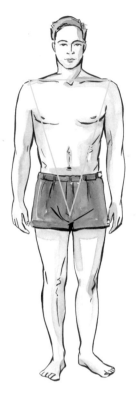
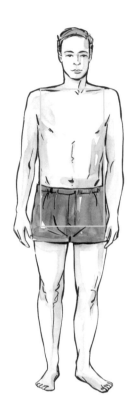
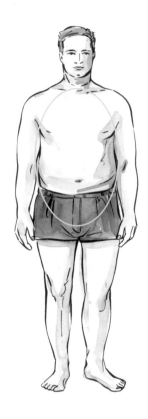
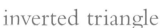

inverted triangle

Broad shoulders narrowing down to the hips. Any Italian styling with its wide lapels and shoulder lines will enhance his body shape – don't hide his athletic silhouette. Choose a crisp, lightweight fabric; any patterns should be geometric or striped. If he is short in the leg, make sure that his trousers are not too wide.

rectangle

Shoulders and hips in line with each other. Standard single or double-breasted British-cut suits will work well if your groom has this body shape – make sure the jacket is slighted waisted – as will all formal occasion wear. Just check his proportions and make sure his jacket sits well against his shirt collar and that the sleeves are the right length.

round

Rounded shoulder line and fuller stomach. The fabric of his outfit needs to be soft to ensure the correct fit across the chest and stomach. If he has a particularly full stomach and his trousers tend to slip below it, consider persuading him into wearing a waistcoat/vest to give a smooth and contoured look to his shape.

men's outfits

THERE ARE DIFFERENT STYLES OF FORMAL WEDDING ATTIRE FOR MEN, SOME OF WHICH ARE MORE TRADITIONAL THAN OTHERS. WHATEVER THE STYLE, IF YOU WEAR A LONG WEDDING GOWN THE MEN'S SUITS SHOULD BE WORN WITH A FORMAL SHIRT AND TIE.

formal styles

Morning dress (tails) This is the most formal suit worn during the day and works well for all body shapes and sizes. It is available in black or charcoal worn with pinstripe trousers or grey worn with matching trousers.

Black tie (tuxedo) Another formal look for weddings held later in the day and for evening receptions. The suit can be either single or double breasted. Choose a revers collar for inverted triangle and rectangle body shapes, a shawl collar for round. For a less formal look, you have the option of adding a coloured tie and waistcoat or cummerbund.

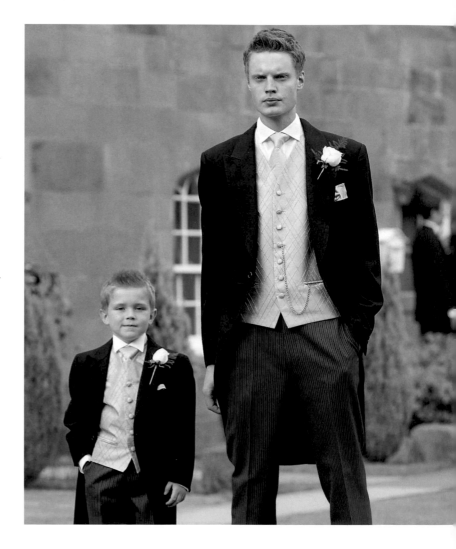

RIGHT *This classic tailcoat is given an updated look with a fashionable silk waistcoat and matching tie.*

Frock coat A recent popular addition to the wedding scene, the frock coat can be made from luxury fabrics such as brocade or velvet. It is best suited to average to tall inverted triangle and rectangle body shapes, but can be worn with a waistcoat by a tall, round man.

Lounge suit This is the most relaxed of formal wear and is suitable for any time of day. If the men aren't used to wearing suits during the day, this might be their most comfortable option. Choose fabrics carefully: a crisper fabric for an inverted triangle, lightweight worsted for a rectangle and a softer, woven fabric such as lightweight flannel for a round body shape.

alternatives

If a uniform is part of your groom's life, he may wear the formal version of it for your wedding. The same applies if he has a traditional dress, religious or otherwise. For an informal wedding, you may want him in a lounge suit, with or without a tie. A tropical wedding calls for a white dinner jacket.

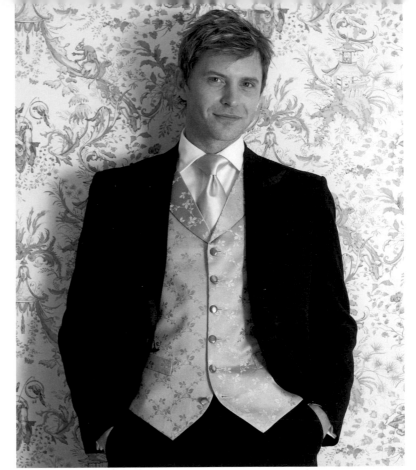

on view too

Whether you want the best man, fathers and ushers (groomsmen) to wear the same as the groom is entirely a personal choice. However, the best man usually wears the same style of suit as the groom. What the other men in the bridal party wear often depends on the formality of the wedding.

If you choose to have a page boy (or ring bearer), just make sure that he is comfortable in what he wears to avoid any last-minute tantrums.

ABOVE *The formality of the black tie has been given a wedding makeover with a silk waistcoat and tie.*

HIRING

Don't hesitate to hire the men's attire, but make sure that they have all tried their suits on in advance and that sleeve lengths are correct and trousers fit properly.

men's accessories

THE WAY THE MEN IN THE BRIDAL PARTY WEAR THE VARIOUS ACCESSORIES THAT COMPLETE THEIR OUTFIT IS IMPORTANT, AND YOU WILL WANT TO MAKE SURE THEY GET IT RIGHT. THIS IS WHERE YOU CAN CO-ORDINATE OR CONTRAST COLOURS, AND ALLOW THE GROOM TO DEMONSTRATE SOME OF HIS PERSONALITY.

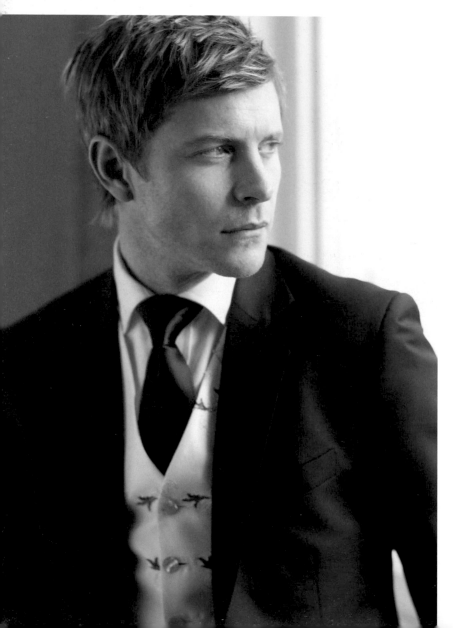

shirts, ties and cufflinks

The choice of shirt will depend on the choice of neckwear:

Tie A standard tie requires a standard shirt collar.

Self-tie cravat or scrunchy This can be worn with a standard or wing collar.

Cravat A cravat dictates a wing collar to go with it.

Bow tie Team this with a standard or wing collar. Whatever the type of neckwear, it must be made from silk so that it falls well.

Cufflinks These are only worn with a shirt that has double (French) fold back cuffs. Beware of choosing jokey inappropriate cufflinks for a formal wedding.

LEFT *A colour co-ordinated waistcoat and tie turn a lounge suit into something special.*

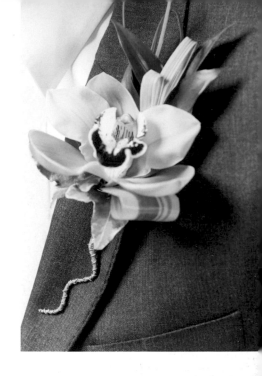

waistcoats

You can choose a waistcoat in the same colour as the jacket or a contrasting one. Consider having the groom wear something different from the rest of the men in order for him to stand out and make his own fashion statement! With any waistcoat, always leave the lowest button open.

cummerbunds, belts and braces

A cummerbund can be worn with a black tie (tuxedo) and is great for tidying up the waist line and disguising a rounded stomach. A cummerbund should always be teamed with a bow tie, and you can have fun choosing a suitable colour for both.

If the suit trousers have loops, these call for a belt (and certainly no braces). If the suit is hired and is unable to be altered to fit for the occasion and there are no belt loops, braces will be needed.

Under no circumstances should any of these three be worn together.

grooming

Just like you, your partner needs to think about his grooming in advance of the day.

Make sure he has booked a haircut that will look just right in time for the photographs. If he has heavy brows, they should be controlled – you may need to get out your tweezers. It goes without saying that shaving or beard trimming must be attended to at the appropriate time prior to the ceremony. The groom's hands will also be on display on the day, so treat him to a manicure the day before the wedding or do it yourself if you have time.

shoes and socks

Black shoes should be highly polished and not scuffed; black patent can be worn with black tie. Make sure any labels on the soles are removed before wearing them.

Socks should be worn in plain, dark colours and made from wool, cotton or silk. Avoid man-made fibres to prevent discomfort. They should be long enough to cover the lower calf.

ABOVE *A colourful buttonhole easily co-ordinates with the rest of the bridal party.*

boutonnières (buttonholes)

A boutonnière is a small flower arrangement for the buttonhole. Your groom's boutonnière should relate in variety of flowers and/or colour to your own bouquet.

Boutonnières for the rest of the men in the bridal party should be in the style or colour of the groom's, but not exactly the same in other respects. Make sure that the stem of the boutonnière is securely pinned to the lapel.

mothers' outfits

YOUR WEDDING DAY IS ALSO A MOMENTOUS ONE IN YOUR MOTHER'S LIFE, AND YOUR FUTURE MOTHER-IN-LAW'S, TOO. YOU WILL WANT THEM TO BE HAPPY AND RELAXED ON THE DAY, AND WHAT THEY WEAR IS VERY MUCH PART OF HOW THEY WILL FEEL — NOT TO MENTION LOOKING GOOD IN THE PHOTOGRAPHS!

fitting in

Both mothers should wait until you have selected your own dress and those of your bridesmaids before choosing their own, so that they too can feel part of the bridal party and neither under- nor over-dressed.

colours

The mothers may want to bring some of your colour theme into their own outfits, perhaps in a trim, an accessory or even a corsage. What you want to avoid is a kaleidoscope of colours made up of your dress, your bridesmaids' and the mothers' – unless that is specifically the effect you are trying to create.

For more detailed advice on colours, see pages 12–17.

RIGHT *This three-piece outfit co-ordinates with the hat and colourful shoes for a special event.*

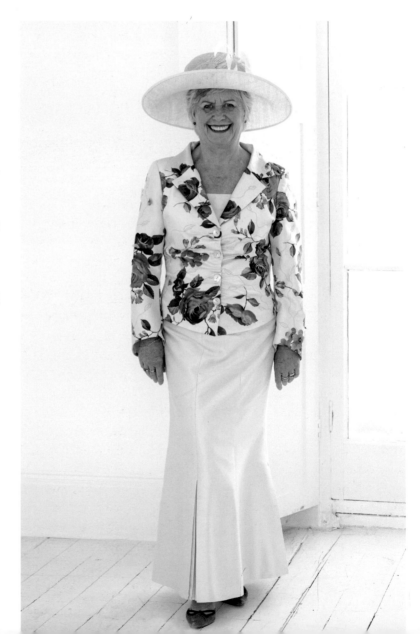

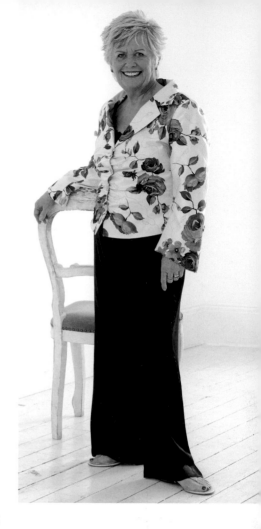

To ensure they choose the best colours to complement their colourings, why not treat both mothers to a **colour me beautiful** colour consultation?

style

The style of the mothers' outfits will depend on the style of your wedding, the time of the year and when it is taking place.

This will probably be one of the most expensive outfits they will ever buy. To make it a more economical purchase, they should consider its practicalities and whether there will be occasions in the future when they can wear it again. For example, an elaborate outfit could be worn at other formal occasions (dinner dances); a simple outfit, such as a shift dress and coat, could be accessorized with a fabulous hat and shoes for the wedding, and thereafter worn more simply for a graduation, christening or work-related event and accessorized accordingly.

Other options are to buy an outfit that can be altered after the event to make it more useful: say, by shortening a long dress or skirt that can then be worn for less formal occasions. One of the most versatile 'mother of the bride' outfits is a three-piece suit, which can then be split into the three different pieces to be worn with the rest of her wardrobe.

shoes and handbags

The mothers' shoes must be comfortable and, just like yours, should be worn around the house to break them in. They should be in a style that they have worn before so that they are used to walking and standing around in them.

Make sure your mother's handbag is big enough to take what she needs to carry for herself and, perhaps, you – and don't forget the tissues.

make-up

The wedding will be an emotional day for your mother, so make sure her make-up is long lasting; waterproof mascara is a good precaution against smudged make-up.

MIX, NOT MATCH

When shopping for a mother's outfit, you do not necessarily have to announce to the store assistants that you are looking for a wedding outfit – unless you want her to come out dressed in matching fabric from head to toe.

mothers' hats

face shape

Before selecting a hat with your mother, remember that her face shape may have changed over the years. It might be fuller, or thinner than it was twenty years ago.

Oval Any shape of hat can be worn and should be placed straight across the brow.

Square Asymmetric shapes are good, worn slightly tilted.

Rectangle A hat with a brim and flatter crown, worn straight or tilted, is best.

Inverted triangle Avoid hats with a large brim and choose slightly softer lines rather than dramatic asymmetric ones.

Round Rounded crowns and brims work better than straight ones, and should be worn at a slight angle.

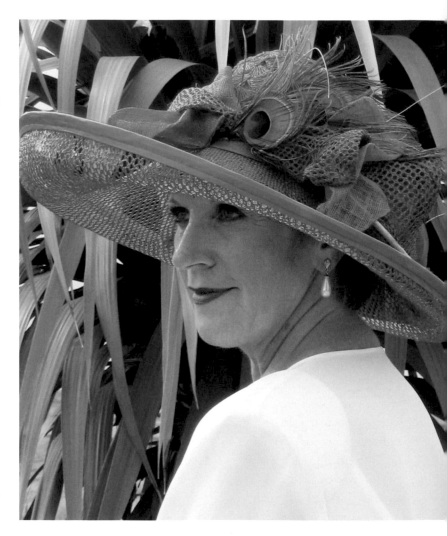

RIGHT *A contrasting colourful hat will set off a neutral outfit beautifully.*

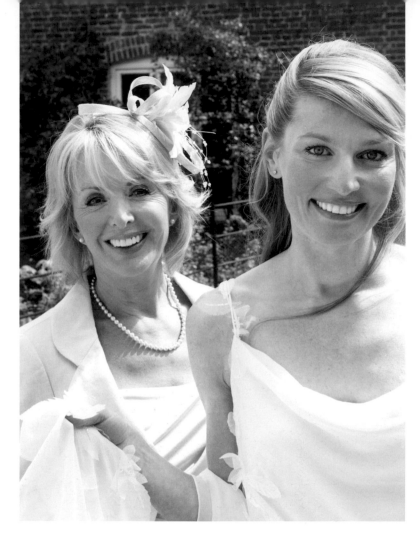

colour

A matching hat and outfit will always look contrived and give the impression that the wearer has no imagination. Conversely, a complementary or contrasting colour will bring interest to the outfit. Be aware that black or dark colours will cast dark shadows over the face and these will show on the photographs.

LEFT *A pretty feather fascinator will not disturb your mother's hairstyle.*

FASCINATORS

If a hat fills your mother with dread, a fascinator (see pages 84–85) is a fashionable alternative. If your wedding is an all-day event, a fascinator will not mess up her hair and she won't collide into other hats when kissing their wearers. The fascinator can be as simple or as extravagant as desired – remember that it will not necessarily be a cheaper option than a hat. It is attached to the head with a comb or invisible elastic and should be positioned carefully to complement your mother's face shape, proportions and hairstyle.

size

First, take note of height and scale: a petite woman will be overwhelmed by a large hat, while a small hat will be lost on a larger-scale woman. The brim of the hat should not extend beyond the shoulders, and the crown should not be narrower than the cheekbones. If your mother is petite in height, consider a hat with a taller crown.

shape

A straight or up-turned brim will give a lift to the face, while a brim that slopes down will cast shadows over it and emphasize heavy jaws, and is not good on a short neck. Make sure the line of the hat complements the line of your mother's clothes. Softer-styled hats work well with softer, fluid clothes, asymmetric hats with straight lines and constructed outfits.

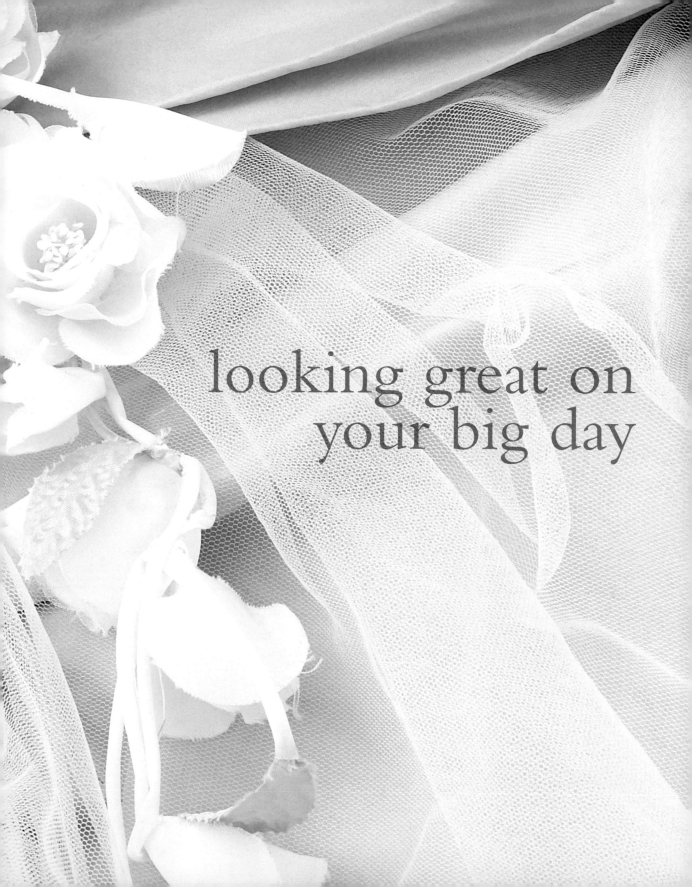

looking great on
your big day

bridal lingerie

THIS IS THE DAY ON WHICH SPECIAL UNDERWEAR IS CALLED FOR. DON'T JUST RUSH OUT AND BUY A NEW SET OF THE THINGS YOU NORMALLY WEAR: YOUR LINGERIE NEEDS TO WORK WITH THE STYLE OF WEDDING DRESS YOU ARE GOING TO WEAR. DO NOT BE SHY ABOUT TAKING ADVICE FROM THE PROFESSIONALS.

colours and textures

Check how fine or translucent the fabric of your dress is before choosing embellished, lacy underwear. Flesh-coloured lingerie shows far less through whites or creams than pure white, which will stand out against your skin, particularly if you are tanned. With other colours of wedding dress, have fun co-ordinating the shades.

bras

You will need to be measured properly before you buy a bra. Brand sizes vary and you will even find that different shapes of bra call for different-sized cups. Once properly fitted, your bra will be comfortable yet give you support, so there should

RIGHT *Every bride deserves beautiful underwear under her dress.*

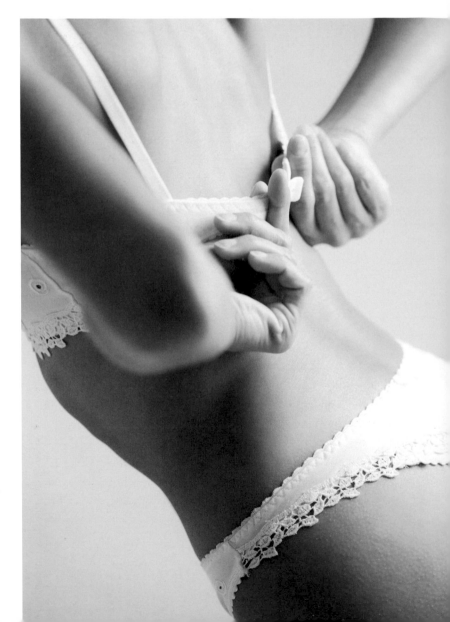

116

be no need for you to tug, pull or fidget with it on the day.

If you are wearing a corset- or bustier-style bodice, you may not need any further support as the garment is fitted to you. You may want to wear a bustier under your dress, so make sure it is comfortable and there are no bones or wiring cutting into you, especially when you sit down.

If your wedding dress has sleeves, you might like to have little ribbons sewn in on the shoulders to prevent your bra straps wandering.

panties

No Visible Pantie Line, please. You may be tempted to put yourself into 'magic' high-control knickers – just make sure you have worn them in advance and are comfortable with what they do to your body. A good alternative is an all-in-one body shaper. If your dress is sheer and you feel comfortable in bikini-style panties or a thong, these can provide the solution to a VPL.

Whatever you choice, make sure you are able to answer nature's calls easily.

hosiery

Brides are often tempted to wear hold-ups or stockings on their wedding day rather than tights, which do not have much sex appeal. If you go for stockings and your skirt is slim fitting, make sure the clasps on your suspender belt are covered with ribbon.

If you have chosen open shoes, wear hosiery with vision heels and toes.

petticoats

The style of your dress will dictate what petticoat, if any, you need to wear in order for it to fall properly. For example, a ballgown style will invariably come with layers and layers of petticoats, while an A-line dress may need one to stiffen up the line a little, if that is the look you are after.

The supplier of your dress will be able to show you a variety of petticoats best suited to your dress. Shifts or empire-line dresses are unlikely to need petticoats as they should already be fully lined. If they are not, you will need a simple slip under the dress to ensure it hangs without clinging.

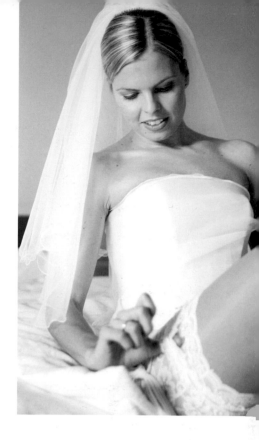

ABOVE *Wearing the right underwear will ensure you are comfortable all day long.*

TIPS FOR THE DAY

Make sure you try the complete set of underwear with your dress to ensure there are no see-through VPL or other unsightly lumps and bumps. Wear the underwear for a day to make certain it is practical and comfortable, whether standing up or sitting down.

getting ready

WHETHER YOU ARE A MAKE-UP *AFICIONADO* OR HAVE NEVER TOUCHED THE STUFF, ON YOUR WEDDING DAY YOU MUST BE PREPARED TO MAKE SOME CHANGES TO YOUR STANDARD ROUTINE. YOUR MAKE-UP WILL NEED TO LAST FOR THE DURATION OF THE EVENT, SO SPECIAL APPLICATION MAY BE NECESSARY. YOU MAY CHOOSE TO HAVE YOUR MAKE-UP DONE FOR YOU – JUST MAKE SURE YOUR GROOM WILL RECOGNIZE YOU AS YOU WALK DOWN THE AISLE. REHEARSING HOW YOU WILL LOOK ON THE DAY IS A MUST.

application techniques

A good skincare routine is essential and should have started some months before the wedding. On the day, make sure you allow enough time before the photographer arrives to apply your make-up or have it applied to you.

Skin Prepare your skin with a primer, which helps to even out your complexion and ensure that your foundation lasts longer. Apply foundation with a sponge or brush, working one area at a time rather than dotting it around. Next, if necessary, apply concealer to hide any blemishes or dark circles. Using a large powder puff or cotton wool, powder the whole of your face, avoiding the eye area, and then powder again.

The layers will give a long-lasting finish to your make-up. Remove any excess with a powder brush.

Eyes Use an eye base on your eyelids to prevent your eye shadows creasing. Apply mascara generously, leaving time for it to dry between coats and concentrating on the outer edge – on your wedding day, a waterproof mascara is a must. Use a pencil if your eyebrows require definition.

Lips Lip base forms the perfect starting point for your lip colour application, which should be followed by lip pencil. Apply lipstick/gloss with a lip brush. Use a single layer of tissue over the lips and then powder over with your brush. Finally, gently spray your whole face with a fine water mist.

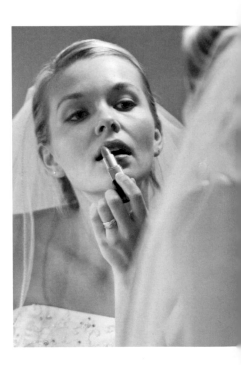

ABOVE *Layering your lipstick will ensure a long lasting application.*

light make-up colours

THE OVERALL LOOK OF YOUR MAKE-UP WILL BE LIGHT AND DELICATE, SO DO NOT OVERPOWER IT WITH STRONG, DARK SHADES FOR EITHER EYE SHADOWS OR LIPSTICK.

EYE SHADOW

CHAMPAGNE   PEACH   AQUA   MELON   LAVENDER BLISS   GOLD WHISPER

EYE PENCIL

COFFEE   GRANITE   TEAL

LIPSTICK / GLOSS

TULIP   CORAL   TOPAZ   DUSTY ROSE   SILK   ALFRESCO

LIP PENCIL

NATURAL   SPICE   CANTALOUPE

BLUSHER

SALMON   CANDY   MARSALA

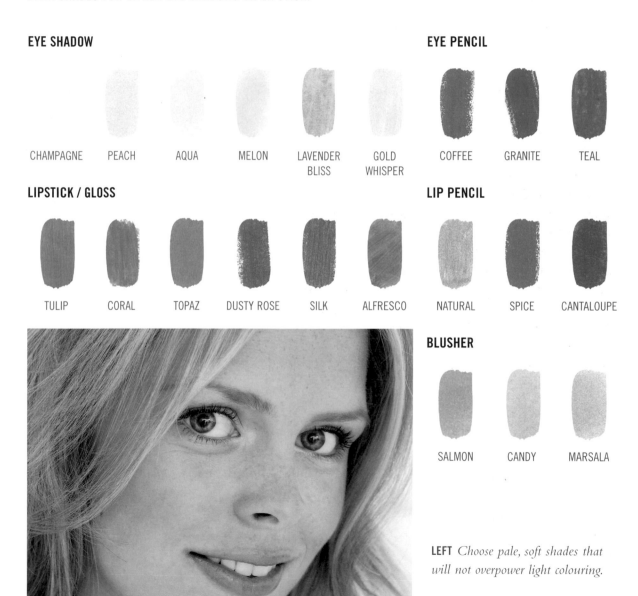

LEFT *Choose pale, soft shades that will not overpower light colouring.*

deep make-up colours

ALTHOUGH YOUR COLOURING IS DEEP, ON YOUR WEDDING DAY YOUR MAKE-UP NEEDS TO BE A LITTLE LIGHTER THAN YOU WOULD NORMALLY WEAR. GO FOR STRONG EYES AND LIGHTER LIPS OR VICE VERSA.

EYE SHADOW

APRICOT TOFFEE COCOA HEATHER KHAKI BAYLEAF

EYE PENCIL

SOFT BLACK PETROL BROWN

LIPSTICK / GLOSS

KAZZBAR MAHOGANY RUBY RUM SAVANNAH TAMARIND

LIP PENCIL

RED RUSSET SPICE

BLUSHER

COGNAC PORT MUSCAT

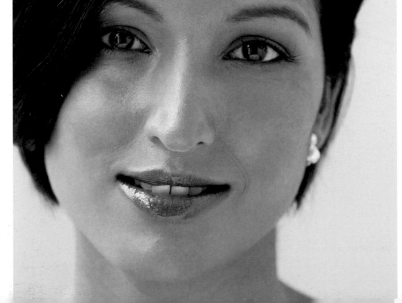

RIGHT *Defining eyes with a pencil gives a dramatic look for a deep bride's colouring.*

warm make-up colours

WHEN CHOOSING YOUR MAKE-UP COLOURS, THINK GOLDEN, COPPER, BRONZE AND AMBER. MAKE SURE THE SHINE AND GLITTER IS KEPT TO A MINIMUM SO THAT THE PHOTOGRAPHER'S FLASH DOESN'T REFLECT TOO MUCH.

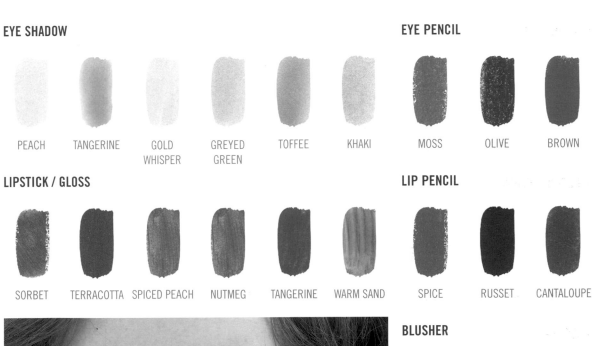

EYE SHADOW

PEACH · TANGERINE · GOLD WHISPER · GREYED GREEN · TOFFEE · KHAKI

EYE PENCIL

MOSS · OLIVE · BROWN

LIPSTICK / GLOSS

SORBET · TERRACOTTA · SPICED PEACH · NUTMEG · TANGERINE · WARM SAND

LIP PENCIL

SPICE · RUSSET · CANTALOUPE

BLUSHER

COGNAC · ALMOND · SALMON

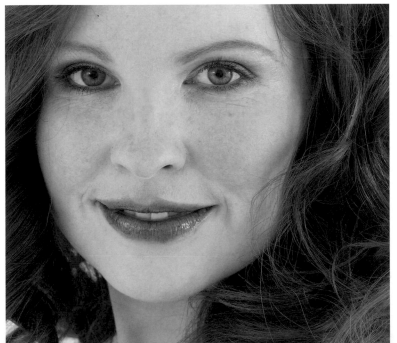

LEFT *All this warm bride's make-up shades have a hint of gold or yellow in them.*

cool make-up colours

YOUR ROSY COMPLEXION AND COOL EYES WILL BE COMPLEMENTED BY COOL SHADES. BLENDING YOUR EYE SHADOWS TOGETHER WILL ENSURE YOUR EYES SHINE THROUGHOUT THE DAY.

EYE SHADOW

| OPAL | PEARL | MERCURY | DELPH | DUSK | HEATHER | MARINE | AMETHYST | GRANITE |

EYE PENCIL

LIPSTICK / GLOSS

| BONBON | CERISE | SOFT MAUVE | PINK SHELL | FUCHSIA | SANGRIA | ROSE | POSIE | NATURAL |

LIP PENCIL

BLUSHER

| ROSE | PORT | CANDY |

RIGHT *Soft pink lipstick and blusher bring out the colour in this cool bride's eyes.*

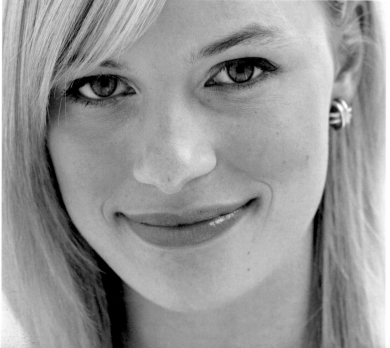

clear make-up colours

BRIGHT, CLEAR COLOURS AS EITHER LIPSTICK OR EYE SHADOW ARE A MUST TO CREATE YOUR WEDDING MAKE-UP.
JUST LIKE YOU, IT MUST BE STRIKING.

EYE SHADOW

CHAMPAGNE	PEPPERMINT	STEEL	LAGOON	INDIAN OCEAN	TANGERINE

EYE PENCIL

PETROL	AMETHYST	SOFT BLACK

LIPSTICK / GLOSS

WARM PINK	FIESTA	STRAWBERRY	MANGO	ALFRESCO	CORAL

LIP PENCIL

RED	CANTALOUPE	POSIE

BLUSHER

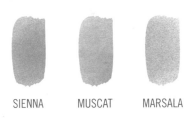

SIENNA	MUSCAT	MARSALA

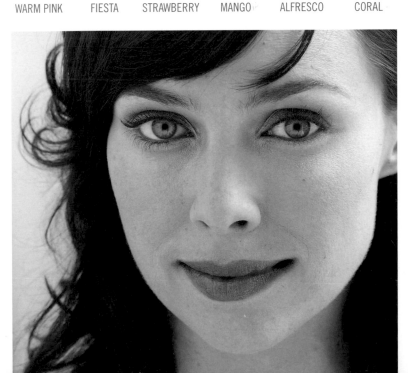

LEFT *This clear bride's stunning blue eyes are perfectly complemented with a bright lipstick.*

soft make-up colours

YOUR GENTLE, SOFT EYES SHOULD NOT BE OVERPOWERED BY BRIGHT-COLOURED SHADOWS AND PENCILS. DO NOT
FORGET THAT IF YOUR EYEBROWS ARE BLONDE THEY MAY REQUIRE A LITTLE DEFINITION.

EYE SHADOW

MELON   FAWN   PEWTER   SMOKE   INDIAN OCEAN   LILAC   COCOA   MOSS   AUBERGINE

EYE PENCIL

LIPSTICK / GLOSS

SANDALWOOD   SOFT MAUVE   BREEZE   NUDE   WARM SAND   PINK SHELL   NATURAL   SPICE   ROSE

LIP PENCIL

BLUSHER

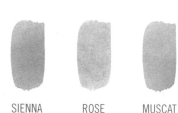

SIENNA   ROSE   MUSCAT

RIGHT *Blended smoky eyes work
wonderfully well with natural toned
lipstick for this soft bride.*

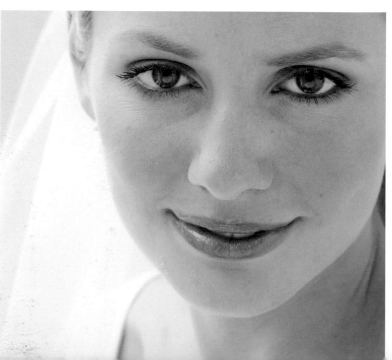

final word

grooming

Your grooming schedule should begin two to three months before the big day. By the time your wedding arrives you should have established a good skincare routine, your body should be waxed and, if necessary, eyebrows should have been shaped and tinted, as well as your eyelashes. Treat yourself to a couple of pedicures and manicures before the day.

if you wear glasses

You may want to consider some options that will fit in well with what you are wearing. If you choose a traditional white dress, dark-framed glasses will over-power the look – rimless glasses or half-frames are better. Non-reflective lenses will ensure your eyes are seen through the lens rather than the flash of the camera bulb.

RIGHT *Careful preparation will ensure you look your best when the day finally arrives.*

emergency kit

Someone in the bridal party will need to take charge of an emergency kit, which should contain a spare pair of tights/stockings as well as sticking plasters (in case you haven't broken in your shoes properly). An emery board and spare needle and thread might also be useful. Don't forget the indigestion tablets, headache pills and tissues.

You should also entrust somone with your make-up bag, which should contain powder, mascara, lip pencil and lipstick/gloss to refresh your look during the day.

good photography

Remember that shimmer and shine in your make-up will grab the light for colour photography, so make sure you keep your make-up matt. Don't forget to eat *before* you start the final countdown to applying your make-up and getting dressed, and it's best to drink through a straw before the ceremony.

You will be asked to smile a thousand times on your wedding day, so a trip to the dental hygienist a week or so before will give you a beaming smile all day.

Have a wonderful wedding day!

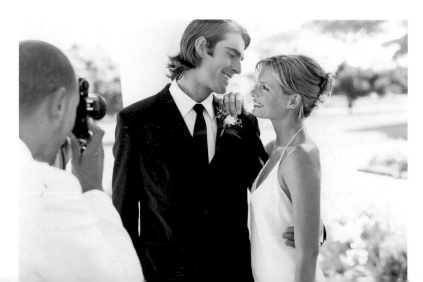

index

Page numbers in italics refer to illustrations.

acknowledgements

This book would not have seen the light of day without Chris Scarles thinking about 350,000 brides whose first thought after the proposal is what they are going to wear.

The Hamlyn team was totally supportive and fun to work with. Jasmine, gardenia and orchid whites now hold no secrets for them.

The critical input of Louise Ravenscroft on the first draft was, as ever, much appreciated.

Christine Southam was particularly generous in handing over her wedding treasure case complete with Ian Stuart dress, while Rose Southam's bridesmaid paraphernalia was also shared with us. Ancilla McPherson also kindly lent us her wedding dress.

Audrey Sirian (just married) advised us of what a bride-to-be would be looking for in this book. Thank you to her photographer, Kelsy Nielson.

The colour me beautiful head office team of Rosalie Poels (newly engaged) and Fiona Wellins were as helpful as usual in organising the dresses and accessories; both are now dab hands at ironing wedding dresses. Thanks too to Georgina Scarles and Sophie Scarles for their help on the busy photoshoot.

Even though we've both been married for some decades, this book brought back many lovely memories. We wish all the brides-to-be and their mothers as much fun as we have had in writing this bridal manual.

Pat Henshaw & Veronique Henderson

Executive Editor Katy Denny
Senior Editor Charlotte Macey
Executive Art Editor Penny Stock
Designer Geoff Borin
Senior Production Controller
  Amanda Mackie
Picture Research
  Zoë Spilberg

Picture acknowledgements

Special photography: © Octopus Publishing Group Limited/Vanessa Davies.

Other photography: Alamy Ace Stock Ltd 71, Chris Rout/Bubbles Photolibrary 72, i love images 103 centre, Image Source Black 98, Jupiter Images/Brand X 92, Ron Chapple Stock 73, Sean Bolton 109, Stockbyte 58; Corbis Elisa Lazo de Valdez 70, Pool Photography 15, Reuters 13, Richard T Nowicz 97 below; Favourbrook Menswear, London 107, 108; Getty Images Andersen Ross/Stockbyte 118, ColorBlind Images 4, Comstock 102 centre, Harald Eisenberger 117, Hitoshi Nishimura 55, Ryan McVay 101, Stephen Wallis 89 above, Stockbyte 102 right; Etiquette at Austin Reed 106; Hats By Sherry www.hatsbysherry.co.uk 112; IPC Syndication all 90–91; istockphoto.com iofoto 103 left; Johanna Hehir 49; photo by Kelsy Nielson 83; Masterfile 97 above; Octopus Publishing Group Mike Prior 104; PA Photos 17, James Whatling/UK Press 40 right, Pressens 12, Robert Evans/AP 41 right; Photolibrary VStock 102 left; Punchstock 125, DAJ 51; Rex Features 14, Action Press 16, Sipa Press 41 left; SuperStock Anton Vengo 103 right; Tips Images Ltd Bildagentur 11, Juice Images 113, Photononstop 116; Vera Mont 69 www.veramont.com

---

Many thanks to the following for providing dressses, shoes, flowers and accessories for the photoshoot:

DRESSES
alfredangelo.com
bhs.co.uk
foreverbridal.com
ianstuart-bride.com
motasem.co.uk
pronovias.com

SHOES
victoriaallinson.co.uk
lkbennett.co.uk

FLOWERS
Georgie Bailey Floral Design:
www.gbfd.co.uk

ACCCESSORIES
Luellasboudoir.co.uk
Yarwood-white.com

Please contact Colour Me Beautiful for more information on services, products and how to become a consultant:

UK and Headquarters for Europe, Africa and the Middle East
66 The Business Centre,
15–17 Ingate Place,
London SW8 3NS
www.colourmebeautiful.co.uk
info@cmb.co.uk
+44 (0)20 7627 5211

China
www.qixincolor.com
Finland
www.colourmebeautiful.fi
Ireland
www.cmbireland.com
Hong Kong
www.colourmebeautiful.hk

Netherlands, Germany & Belgium
www.colourmebeautiful.nl
Norway
www.colour-me-beautiful.no
Portugal
www.cmb.com.pt
Slovenia
www.cmb.si
South Africa
www.colormebeautiful.co.za
Spain
www.colourmebeautiful.es
Sweden
www.colourmebeautiful.se
USA
www.colormebeautiful.com